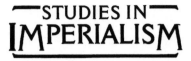

STUDIES IN IMPERIALISM

General editor: Andrew S. Thompson
Founding editor: John M. MacKenzie

When the 'Studies in Imperialism' series was founded more than twenty-five years ago, emphasis was laid upon the conviction that 'imperialism as a cultural phenomenon had as significant an effect on the dominant as on the subordinate societies'. With well over a hundred titles now published, this remains the prime concern of the series. Cross-disciplinary work has indeed appeared covering the full spectrum of cultural phenomena, as well as examining aspects of gender and sex, frontiers and law, science and the environment, language and literature, migration and patriotic societies, and much else. Moreover, the series has always wished to present comparative work on European and American imperialism, and particularly welcomes the submission of books in these areas. The fascination with imperialism, in all its aspects, shows no sign of abating, and this series will continue to lead the way in encouraging the widest possible range of studies in the field. 'Studies in Imperialism' is fully organic in its development, always seeking to be at the cutting edge, responding to the latest interests of scholars and the needs of this ever-expanding area of scholarship.

Beyond the state

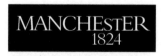

MANCHESTER
1824

Manchester University Press

Beyond the state

THE COLONIAL MEDICAL SERVICE IN BRITISH AFRICA

Edited by Anna Greenwood

MANCHESTER
UNIVERSITY PRESS

Published by Manchester University Press
Altrincham Street, Manchester M1 7JA
www.manchesteruniversitypress.co.uk

British Library Cataloguing-in-Publication Data
A catalogue record for this book is available from the British Library

Library of Congress Cataloging-in-Publication Data applied for

ISBN   978 0 7190 8967 1   hardback

First published 2016

Typeset by
Servis Filmsetting Ltd, Stockport Cheshire
Printed in Great Britain by
TJ International Ltd, Padstow

CONTENTS

[v]

NOTES ON CONTRIBUTORS

Shane Doyle is Senior Lecturer in African History at the University of Leeds. His publications on the history of demography, environmental change, ethnicity, medicine and sexuality include two monographs, *Crisis and Decline in Bunyoro: Population and Environment in Western Uganda 1860–1955* (Oxford, James Currey and Athens OH, Ohio University Press, 2006) and *Before HIV: Sexuality, Fertility and Mortality in East Africa, 1900–1980* (London, British Academy and Oxford University Press, 2013). He has also edited a collected volume with Henri Médard, *Slavery in the Great Lakes Region of East Africa* (Ohio University Press, 2007).

Anna Greenwood is Assistant Professor in the History of British Imperialism at the University of Nottingham. She has published widely on the history of the Colonial Medical Service in Africa, medical impressions of the African climate and the theoretical uses of history in other social science disciplines. She has two monographs, *Practising Colonial Medicine: The Colonial Medical Service in British East Africa* (London, I.B. Tauris, 2007 [under the name of Crozier]) and with Harshad Topiwala, *Indian Doctors in Kenya: The Forgotten Story, 1895–1940* (Palgrave Macmillan, 2015).

Matthew M. Heaton is Assistant Professor in the Department of History at Virginia Tech. His research interests revolve around the intersections of nationalism, globalisation, and health in twentieth century Nigeria. He is the author of *Black Skin, White Coats: Nigerian Psychiatrists, Decolonization, and the Globalization of Psychiatry* (Athens OH, Ohio University Press, 2013), and the co-author of *A History of Nigeria* (Cambridge, Cambridge University Press, 2008). He is also the author of several articles and book chapters as well as co-editor of several volumes on health and illness in African history.

Markku Hokkanen is a Docent and Senior Lecturer at the Department of History and Ethnology, University of Jyväskylä. His research deals with the cultural, social and intellectual histories of medicine and health in the modern era, with a focus on colonial Africa (particularly Malawi) and the British Empire. His publications include *Medicine and Scottish Missionaries in the Northern Malawi Region, 1875–1930* (The Edwin Mellen Press, 2007) and 'Imperial Networks, Colonial Bioprospecting and Burroughs Wellcome & Co' (*Social History of Medicine*, 25, 3,

2012). Hokkanen's current research interests are mobility, networks and the making of medical knowledge in the imperial age.

Michael Jennings is Senior Lecturer in International Development at SOAS, University of London. He is also Chair of the Centre of African Studies, University of London. Michael has published widely on the history of development in East Africa, linking historical themes into contemporary development practice and theory. His work has a particular focus on the role of non-state actors (especially non-governmental organisations, faith-based organisations and missionary societies) in development and service delivery, and their relations with states, donors and the communities in which they work. He also writes on historical and contemporary issues relating to health and healing in Africa.

Yolana Pringle is a Mellon-Newton Postdoctoral Research Fellow at the University of Cambridge. Her research interests include the history of psychiatry and mental health, humanitarian intervention, and East African social history. She has published articles in the *Journal of the History of Medicine and Allied Sciences* and the *Journal of Imperial and Commonwealth History*, and is currently writing a monograph on the development of mental health care in Uganda.

Harshad Topiwala is an Honorary Research Fellow at the School of History in the University of Kent, UK. He has a keen interest in the history of the British Empire and has actively researched colonial medicine for a decade. The findings have been presented in a number of international conferences and the research published in a monograph (with Anna Greenwood), *Indian Doctors in Kenya: The Forgotten Story, 1895–1940* (Palgrave Macmillan, 2015). Harshad has lived and worked in a number of countries as a senior executive employed by the multinational oil company Shell. He has also been a non-executive Board member, Vice Chair and Chair of NHS Trusts in the UK.

ACKNOWLEDGEMENTS

This book is very much a group effort and without the insights provided by its contributors it would certainly not have come to fruition. Where authors have wanted to thank individuals for providing support they have had the opportunity to do so at the end of their chapter. As the general editor I personally would like to extend my particular thanks to Ryan Johnson for providing the impetus to start this book and for acting as a very good sounding board for its ideas. I also thank my colleagues within the sub-discipline of medical history, many of whom, whether they know it or not (!), directly helped to further my ideas for this book through their ever-incisive questioning. In this regard, I would like to particularly thank Sanjoy Bhattacharya, Pratik Chakrabarti and Jim Mills. My grateful thanks are extended too to the anonymous reviewer of this manuscript; they provided fabulously useful and constructive feedback and this book is very much improved directly because of their astute commentary. I also want to say a collective thank you to all the staff at MUP who made the production of this book possible, as well as the numerous librarians and archivists that assisted me over the past couple of years. I am very proud that all of the papers presented in this book are the result of fresh archival research and I genuinely feel that, both collectively and individually, they offer timely advances in our understanding of colonial medical history.

Finally, on a personal note, I thank David Greenwood who, as well as being my lovely Dad, is surely my shrewdest, yet most supportive, academic critic. I dedicate this book to him as well as to the entirely wonderful Sarb and the ever-witty Otto. These exceptional individuals comprise my precious family and make my life immeasurably richer every day through their unfailing love and good humour.

CHAPTER ONE

Introduction: looking beyond the state

Anna Greenwood

There is no fresh news in stating that the history of colonial medicine has changed considerably in the last seventy-five years. As academic interests have expanded, attention has moved away from triumphalist accounts of the conquest of disease in former European colonies to a more critical, less ethno-centric and more socially inclusive examination of the complex relationships between colonial states and colonised societies. Yet, despite much self-congratulation at achieving a comparatively nuanced understanding of these relationships, glaring gaps remain and there is work still to be done. Although certain colonial institutions and policies have been revisited and reassessed by historians in recent times, others still await the benefits of renewed academic consideration. It is the central rationale of this book that the Colonial Medical Service is one of these institutions, and that the time has come for its history to benefit from new eyes and new perspectives.

When my book, *Practising Colonial Medicine*, on the East African Colonial Medical Service was published in 2007, I was sure that I had captured something of the ethos and experience of the cohort of 424 British government doctors that served in Kenya, Uganda and Tanganyika between 1890 and 1939.[1] It soon became apparent, however, that my researches had uncovered only a small slice, barely a sliver, of a much more complicated story. To start with, it quickly became clear that the Colonial Medical Service in Africa was far from the all-white institution that I had portrayed.[2] Additionally, it was not merely the obedient handmaiden of the British government, but sometimes functioned within its peripheral African locations independently of British command. When colonial officers or governors sought guidance, they were as likely to do so by consulting the precedents established in other colonial possessions – within and outside the African continent – as they were to appeal to the politicians and bureaucrats residing in their mother country. Furthermore, the financially stretched

Colonial Medical Service in Africa rarely acted entirely autonomously; in fact, resources and expertise with other locally functioning health agencies were often formally or informally pooled. For sure, there was not always accord and agreement between different groups working under different masters, but facilities and resources were scarce and pragmatism often overcame institutional separatism.

As I scratched beneath the surface, all sorts of preconceptions fell away. This was a state institution with centralised policies, and with a certain public face to maintain, but nevertheless its members did not speak with one voice, were not of one colour and were not uniformly obedient. Moreover, colonial medical officers often worked closely with groups whose objectives might be conceived as being in competition with the British government. By talking about officers' shared experiences, backgrounds and attitudes in my 2007 monograph I risked falling into the trap of perpetuating exactly the image of unity that the British colonial state would have had the external world believe, rather than exposing the much more complex, and certainly less coherent, reality.

The present volume should be regarded not as an end point but as a starting point from which to think outside the boxes of state and non-state actors. It offers an academic springboard from which to move away from the compartmentalisations to which colonial historical debate is prone: black and white, elites and non-elites, heroes and villains, each operating in neatly delineated secular or religious fields. It instead makes some tentative steps to describing just one small aspect of the untidy reality of Empire. The history of an institution such as the Colonial Medical Service, which seems outwardly to represent the pinnacle of an elite government agency, in fact reveals pervasive and persuasive stereotypes (which undoubtedly also represent some aspects of the reality) that are uncomfortably difficult to sustain.

As well as deconstructing the idea of a unified and unidirectional Colonial Service, grouping these eight essays together in one collection also answers recent demands for more comparative studies in the history of medicine, as opposed to the 'single-site' case studies that have hitherto dominated the discipline. Although concentrating only upon British territories in Africa (obviously the Colonial Service operated only in British possessions), the volume presents cases from several disparate territories covering Kenya, Malawi, Nigeria, Tanganyika, Uganda and Zanzibar. The final work that has emerged concentrates mostly upon the East African region because of the expertise of the scholars who were available to contribute. This should by no means compromise the revisionist intentions of this volume, which are applicable to all regions of Africa in which the Colonial Medical Service operated. Indeed, I hope that these local studies will spur specialists in

[2]

other territories to probe deeper into the bureaucratic fictions woven around the British Colonial Services.

The project has synchronic and diachronic objectives, examining tensions *within* the Colonial Medical Service (as demonstrated by my Chapter Four with Harshad Topiwala on Kenya), as well as the relationships forged *externally* with other agencies, for example with local missionary groups (Chapters Two, Three and Eight by Yolana Pringle, Markku Hokkanen and Michael Jennings, respectively), private firms (Chapter Six, Matthew Heaton), or other (non-medical) research agencies (Chapter Seven, Shane Doyle). An example is also given of when it was deemed unacceptable to work with a competing local medical charity, as is the case in my Chapter Five on relations between the Colonial Medical Service and the Indian- and Arab-dominated Zanzibar Maternity Association. While each case study stands alone in displaying some of the multifaceted dynamics of Colonial Medical Service relationships, it is the intention of this volume to offer these diverse narratives of negotiation as a basis through which to work towards a comparative understanding of the Service's overall reality.

This is not a book applauding the old colonial elites. The Colonial Medical Service has generally been perceived historically as an exclusive and privileged institution, but the greater aim of the book is to expose the intricacies within this enduring stereotype rather than to celebrate it. It is clear that in today's historiographical climate it is more fashionable to speak about those who were ruled than their imperial rulers.[3] Yet both sides of the story are needed if we are to arrive at a truly balanced and considered metanarrative. Besides which, as the book amply illustrates, the Colonial Medical Service, once placed under the historical microscope, was far from being as distinct, cohesive or even as elite, as has generally been assumed.[4] To this end, the overarching aim of this volume is to emphasise both the Colonial Medical Service's internal diversity and its far-reaching external connections. It raises a number of pertinent questions for further debate: to what extent did colonial doctors collaborate with other non-state-orientated organisations? How were both clinical and research agendas mapped and managed? To what extent did informal networks sustain the colonial medical project? What do examples of non-cooperation say about the priorities of the Colonial Medical Service specifically and the colonial state more generally?

The Colonial Service

Belying the uncertain, fluid and complex reality of the British Colonial Services that this collection exposes, the conventional bureaucratic description of the 'mother' organisation of all the Services, The Colonial Service, is quite straightforward. The Colonial Service was the personnel section of the Colonial Office, which was the government department in Whitehall, London responsible for administering the British Empire.[5]

The Colonial Service can therefore be rather simply categorised as the 'people' side of the organisational bureaucracy, overseeing recruitment of staff for Empire, their terms and conditions of service and acting as the main negotiator for transfers between the colonies themselves. The Colonial Service had been in existence since 1838, but it was really first shaken up and reorganised under the tenure of Joseph Chamberlain (1836–1914), who acted as Secretary of State to the Colonies between 1895 and 1903.[6] As part of Chamberlain's vision of 'Constructive Imperialism', he prioritised the rationalisation and streamlining of the colonial bureaucracy in Whitehall, which naturally included scrutinising the internal workings of the Colonial Service. Accordingly, Lord Selborne, the then parliamentary Under-Secretary of State was instructed to produce a report detailing the state of the administration. Selborne reported back in 1899 that he found the Colonial Service to be highly deficient and disorganised: not only were there glaring organisational problems inherent to the way business was arranged centrally, but large discrepancies existed between individual colonies in terms of how work was managed, particularly the disparate terms and conditions of employment that were offered.[7]

Progressively, if slowly, the Colonial Service became more centralised. Reforms peaked in the 1930s with the recommendations provided through the findings of the Warren Fisher Committee, and the Colonial Service was formally organised into vocational branches.[8] The Colonial Administrative Service was one of the first to be unified in 1932, followed in 1934 by the Colonial Medical Service. By 1949 there were twenty branches of the Colonial Service representing, among other areas, education, law, nursing, policing, research and forestry. Although this marked the point of formal rationalisation, archives and source materials reveal that in official and public understandings there had been regionally based Colonial Medical Services since the second half of the nineteenth century. In fact, certain geographically contiguous African medical services had already been unified by the time of the centralised recommendations. The West African Medical Staff (WAMS) brought together the medical services of Nigeria, Gold Coast, Sierra Leone and Gambia in 1902 and the East African Medical Service (EAMS) formally united the services of Kenya, Uganda and Tanganyika in 1921.[9] The Warren Fisher reforms therefore should be seen as an ultimate action in bringing together regional services each under a single

[4]

unified vocational umbrella organisation in London that regularised pay scales and terms and conditions of employment.[10]

Although these reforms centralised things from the perspective of Whitehall, the workaday reality was still very much as it had been when Chamberlain came into office in 1895. Communication difficulties and financial restraints (once staff were *in situ* each service was meant to be locally financially self-supporting) exacerbated the gulf between the lofty ideals put forward within the corridors of Whitehall and the practical restraints of those working in the African continent. The net result was that practice on the ground continued to play itself out mostly responsively to local demands throughout the colonial period and most colonial officers operated independently of this myth of bureaucratic centralisation. This is not to say that changes did not occur in the way the colonies were managed in the period between 1880 and 1960. There were certainly instances in which the interventionist hand of central government was very much felt, but this claim is rather an acknowledgement of the relative fluidity and autonomy of space in which, for better or for worse, local colonial governments necessarily operated. Indeed, it was precisely this local freedom that allowed many of the interactions with non-government actors that are described in the pages that follow.

The Colonial Medical Service

In terms of neatly organised institutional narratives, the Colonial Medical Service was the branch of the administration responsible for the health of colonial staff and local populations in each British colony. It was the second-biggest personnel branch of the British Empire, with Colonial Medical Service employees making up nearly a third of all Colonial Service staff.[11] It was Joseph Chamberlain once again who oversaw the first major changes to the Colonial Medical Service, and, notably, one of his first tasks upon becoming Secretary of State for the Colonies was to appoint Patrick Manson (1844–1922) – then regarded as the most eminent tropical medical specialist of the day – to a newly created position of Consulting Physician to the Colonial Office.[12] This showed the priority assigned to the medical services of Empire. Chamberlain realised that without the tool of medicine, conquest and the maintenance of British supremacy would not be tenable long term, especially in the relatively unknown and climatically hostile environments that Africa presented. In order to address directly an evident need to assure the viability and sustainability of the colonial project by sending qualified doctors out to Empire, Chamberlain and Manson oversaw the founding of the London School of Tropical Medicine; the school opened at the Royal Albert Dock in the East End of London in 1899 as a training facility for new recruits to the Colonial Service. To strengthen this initiative, they also led an active campaign to promote tropical medical education (and by implication colonial careers) for aspiring medical graduates.[13]

Perhaps surprisingly, medical recruitment was always something of an uphill battle, especially when compared to the large competitive demand for the general civil service jobs of Empire. The Indian Civil Service, which required candidates to pass a competitive examination before being offered a position, was regarded as particularly esteemed and could command the very brightest and best young graduates. The reputation of the Colonial Medical Services of Empire was somewhat different. A hierarchy of prestige can nevertheless be discerned, with the Sudan Medical Service generally thought to represent the most prestigious posting. Not only did this service seem to offer the best terms and conditions of employment, but it held elite associations with its famously exclusive sister service, the Sudan Political Service.[14] The Indian Medical Service, though not a particularly popular destination for medical graduates, especially before 1914, nevertheless held a position in the hierarchy that made it more popular than all the African medical services, except Sudan.[15] Of the African services, the WAMS offered a pay supplement to compensate officers for living in the challenging climates of Gold Coast, Nigeria, Sierra Leone or Gambia, where malaria and yellow fever presented a constant threat to life; WAMS was upheld as being something of a model of organisational efficiency. The EAMS, which looked after Kenya, Uganda and, post-1919, Tanganyika (present day Tanzania) was very much lower down the pecking order in terms of prestige, although still preferable to the very small medical services of Nyasaland and Northern and Southern Rhodesia.

Of most marked interest for the thematic emphasis of this collection, the story of recruitment to the Colonial Medical Service is revealing of the large gulfs that existed between the face that the British Empire presented to the Western world and the much more diverse reality of the situation in the colonial localities. Readers of some of the first histories of the Colonial Medical Service in Africa could be forgiven for assuming that all of the medical personnel were of European origin, as most of the histories produced in the decade or so after decolonisation focus only upon white experiences. In fact this was far from true. A great diversity of individuals made up the staff of the Colonial Medical Service and most rural Africans would have had no contact with the European medical officer, but would have been seen at a dispensary by a member of the large cohort of African staff who worked in subordinate medical roles throughout the Empire. But even among the elite class of qualified doctors the situation was far from uniform. As Ryan Johnson has shown, until the turn of the twentieth century, black doctors also served within the WAMS, in one case (Gold Coast Colony) even rising to the rank of Chief Medical Officer.[16] Similarly, as Harshad Topiwala and I point out in Chapter Four, the fact that there were nearly twice as many qualified Indian doctors working for the EAMS as there were white doctors has been perplexingly forgotten in historical accounts.

The selective retelling of the history of the Colonial Medical Service, to the exclusion of non-white faces, reflects the preoccupations of the time in which many of these early medical service histories were written. This was a time before the rise of social history and the critical changes within colonial historiography brought about by the analytical reorientations of the subaltern studies school.[17] Moreover, this was precisely the story that the Colonial Office told to itself and to its public. All recruitment to the African services in London was white recruitment and the other doctors and medical personnel that were recruited for jobs were appointed locally, somewhat quietly, away from the official centralised record keeping. The Colonial Service was very strict in its policy of employing only doctors of European parentage to work in Africa; it would not have done to publicise that in the colonies themselves, doctors were also regularly recruited from Goa or Bombay by local agents.[18]

From the London perspective, the Colonial Medical Service was not a particularly desirable career. Initially, this was heavily to do with the way the ponderous machinery of the Colonial Office worked. Up until the First World War (and tacitly afterwards) most appointments were gained through the 'right' social networks. For doctors, many of whom came from solidly middle-class backgrounds, this was a formidable initial hurdle. It was recognised early on, however, by the first Director of Recruitment between 1910 and 1948, Ralph Furse (1887–1973) that a more meritocratic system needed to be introduced. Officially at least, Colonial Service recruitment became decided through introducing the regularised process of asking interested candidates to submit an official application form and then, if deemed suitable, to attend an interview.

Despite this reorientation, the system remained a highly subjective and not entirely transparent process with individual applicants being turned down for their colour, their lack of sporting prowess or apparent signs of mental weakness.[19] Furse, for all his public commitment to stamping out nepotism and regularising application procedures, was a conservative through and through and had firm ideas about the sort of person that it was desirable to recruit. Doctors from all echelons of society could apply, but the archetypal qualities perceived as being associated with the British public school system were routinely put forward as the most desirable skill-set for the job.[20] Suitable recruits were to be athletic, young, adventurous, resilient, independent and patriotic. Furse himself admitted that 'public school training is of more importance than university training in producing the personality and character capable of handling the natives well'.[21] A certain type was chosen for colonial appointments, and that meant not necessarily recruiting the cream of the medical schools:

> I do not think that we need to attract the very best men. Such men are more useful at home. In the colonies we want a good all-round general practitioner with a good physique and a sporting temperament. Higher attainments are not required, and an unfit man for appointment in so far as there is probably no less satisfactory officer than a man who is too good for his job.[22]

This lack of emphasis upon academic standards was made all the more obvious through the absence of an entrance exam to gain access to the African branches of the Colonial Medical Service.

The unattractiveness of a colonial career for most British medical graduates was compounded by the widespread perception that the pay was not competitive. Pay scales remained surprising static throughout the colonial period. For example, in East Africa a new Medical Officer (MO) could expect to be appointed on a basic salary of £400 per annum, a figure that eventually rose after much campaigning by the British Medical Association to £600 in 1939.[23] In terms of take-home salary, then, officers could easily make much more back home in private or local government practice.[24] Conditions in the colonies were known to be harsh, with meagre facilities, and the chance of integrating wives and families was limited. Add to this the ever-present possibility of serious disease (or even death), and it is hardly surprising that the Colonial Medical Service was never an especially popular career choice and faced intermittent recruitment problems throughout its existence.

On the other hand, the career could, for the right sort of person at least, be an attractive and rewarding one. Life was not for the faint-hearted, but even within this difficult environment there were some palpable advantages to be had. Pay was low, but so was the cost of living. MOs could command a large amount of professional independence, often looking after entire regions and thereby enjoying a local status that they could not have hoped to achieve back home.[25] Communications were slow, and, while this might be a cause for frustration, it meant that individuals could operate independently of the watchful eye of the Colonial Office and come up with their own innovative schemes and models of collaboration. MOs had to work with Asians and Africans in innovative ways that would not have been

possible at home – an exposure that arguably influenced as many individuals to become socially and culturally open as it reinforced in others
a deeper commitment to the dominant racist attitudes. While fully
recognising the many racist assumptions that ran throughout government policies, it must nevertheless be acknowledged that the officers
of Empire were an eclectic bunch, many of whom devoted much time
to learning local African languages and invested huge amounts of personal and professional effort into improving clinical care and levels of
public health. Furthermore, individuals with an active interest in tropical medicine could not conceive of being in a better place in which to
experience at first -hand exciting aspects of medical practice that would
have been impossible back in the UK. Suitably motivated individuals
could, and sometimes did, contribute to making important advances in
the emergent field of tropical medicine.

A picture emerges of a colonial bureaucracy that, although not
popular, was clearly keen to present an organised and unified face to
the British public. One of its central problems was, however, that it
was largely impotent to control the day-to-day character of life in the
colonial outposts. However smooth and centralised the organisation
seemed to be in London, the logistical difficulties of ruling somewhere
as infrastructurally undeveloped as Africa were hard to overcome.
Memos and edicts took days, or even weeks, to arrive and the daily
demands of running busy dispensaries alongside the immediate practicalities of controlling epidemic and endemic diseases were so urgent
that even when instructions did arrive, they were often out of date
and impossible to implement. In practice the head of each territory's
medical department (a role variously called Principal Medical Officer,
Director of Medical Services or Director of Medical and Sanitary
Services) ran his department as best he could in accord with the exi-
gencies of the immediate situation. While this could create a sense of
regional fiefdoms with different priorities and little coordinated practice, it also allowed individual medical services to have relatively free
reign as to how they conducted their business. Even if an order came
through from Whitehall, there was considerable leeway for freedom of
interpretation in the field.

This book will highlight the various and colourful ways that the
organisational self-determination was played out within different
British African colonies. In so doing it destabilises the notion of London
as the stable heart of the colonial administration. The chapters in this
book reveal numerous cases of adaptive working, especially in terms
of the way the Colonial Medical Service could be seen to collaborate
with groups deemed to be operating beyond the formal boundaries of
the state. The time for such a study is ripe, as there has been no study

bringing together the varied experiences of the different regionally based Colonial Medical Services in British Africa, and only a handful of specific regional studies.[26] Tellingly, these studies were mostly written shortly after decolonisation and are characterised by the celebratory tones in which they describe the introduction and dissemination of Western medicine as one of the high points of the British colonial encounter. Only a few works published in the late 2000s offer more balanced perspectives.[27]

One of the key insights provided by the chapters in this book is that, in practice, the Colonial Medical Services were extremely adaptive – Janus-faced, even – looking simultaneously towards the very different requirements of London and Africa.

Colonial Service histories, of course, make up only a very small part of the rich historiography of colonial Africa. This terrain is well known, but the present volume fits extremely well within this wider historical perspective by providing an additional dimension to the ever-expanding scope of colonial historical enquiry that has emerged since the 1980s, deconstructing the old grand narratives of progress in favour of more critically engaged assessments of the social and political encounters of British imperialism.[28]

By common consent, Daniel Headrick started the ball rolling in 1981 with a book that famously shifted interests away from hagiographic accounts of hero doctors dispensing philanthropy, instead critically describing colonial medicine as a political and social 'tool' ultimately used as an aid to imperial domination.[29] This opened the sluice gates of academic reappraisal of the topic, with other highly critical accounts following, including some which have now become extremely well known in the field such as the works of Sanjoy Bhattacharya, John Farley, Mark Harrison, Maryinez Lyons, Randall Packard and Megan Vaughan, among others.[30]

This profound change in ways of evaluating the colonial medical encounter went alongside a renewed interest in trying to locate the voices of the colonised peoples. Immediate source material was scarce, but it was possible to map the way in which united actions of resistance and even, sometimes, outright rebellion, very much mediated the way colonial medical policies were enacted.[31] Such studies set the scene for a closer analysis of sectors of society that had traditionally been neglected by historians.[32] In the context of colonial Africa, this meant studying the roles of native intermediaries, subordinates and clerks who had long existed in the shadows of history and were not thought significant enough to warrant attention in their own right.[33]

Increasingly, colonial medicine was no longer academically discussed solely in terms of an elite Western practice foisted willingly or unwillingly on indigenous peoples. Medicine began to be seen as something that was frequently adapted and appropriated by local people who were often seen to pragmatically amalgamate new cultural traditions with their old ones and embrace pluralism. [34] Other studies stressed the multiple international links within the colonial encounter.[35] Particularly, the usefulness of undertaking broader comparative histories began to be more regularly explored. Examination of the interconnectivities of the different British territories replaced the narrow focus on separate territories of Empire, which was newly recognised as a series of highly complicated networks, with people, ideas and practices all regularly exchanged between its different parts.[36]

These fresh insights had the effect of moving scholars away from studying official government medicine when describing the colonial medical encounter. Missionary medicine came under detailed historical analysis;[37] the link between colonial notions of development and the subsequent channels through which modern international health services operated started to be investigated.[38] Success stories that had been unambiguously applauded for decades were reassessed, such as Sanjoy Bhattacharya's reassessment of the WHO smallpox eradication campaign.[39] The scene had been set for exciting new areas of enquiry, a number of which form the basis of this present book.

Contents of the book

The individual chapters that follow add considerably to our understanding of the multiple, sometimes contradictory ways that medicine was enacted in the colonial localities. In Chapter Two Yolana Pringle deals with relations between government and missionary medical services, covering some of the active collaborations that existed between the Church Missionary Society and the Uganda Colonial Medical Service before 1940. Working with the missions was a pragmatic means of filling a gap in state provision while serving the purposes of the missionaries themselves, as it provided an opportunity to extend their evangelising messages and for individuals to extend their professional range and boost their personal incomes. By taking a broadly chronological approach, and using Mengo Hospital at a case study, Pringle maps the way that relations between the state and missionary medical services subtly changed and evolved. She identifies a shift from short-termist and *ad hoc* responses to slightly more formalised, strategic relationships (particularly with regard to the payment for the services of missionary personnel) but ultimately argues for the persistence of an enduring, if fluid, relationship between state and non-state medical provision. Furthermore, although the contributions of the missions

[11]

shaped the character of colonial state medicine in Uganda, in practice, Pringle notes, patients would have been unaware of any formal delineation between state and non-state medical provision.

Leading on from this discussion, in Chapter Three Markku Hokkanen moves the focus of attention to Nyasaland (Malawi) and the relations that existed there between medical service employees and local missions. In contrast to Pringle's story about Uganda, Hokkanen depicts the Malawian context as containing examples of conflict between the missions and the government medical service, as well as of cooperation. Although numerous examples can be found of the way that the two groups shared materials, equipment, personnel and services, Hokkanen argues that they were deeply divided in their attitudinal stances towards their respective organisations. However, although tensions, professional rivalries and conflicts were regularly expressed, in general it was felt better for these to be kept muted.

It is this desire to present a harmonious and united front that also forms the central point of Chapter Four, by Harshad Topiwala and myself. Here, we take a fresh look at the Colonial Medical Service of Kenya and show that, contrary to popular conceptions of this service, there were almost twice as many Indian doctors working for the Colonial Medical Service as Europeans before 1923. To be sure, these doctors were not appointed, nor paid, at the same rank as MOs, and were, rather, designated Assistant or Sub-Assistant Surgeons, but nevertheless they would have regarded themselves as fully qualified doctors (having attended medical schools in India) and performed clinical and administrative duties largely identical to those of their European counterparts. The chapter explores not only why historians of colonial medicine have previously missed this fact, but also why this state of affairs suddenly stopped in the early 1920s. It is, Topiwala and I conclude, necessarily a complex series of reasons, ones that all nevertheless point towards a strong urge within the Colonial Office to present an image of unity and strength. When the Colonial Service was to be opened up, it was felt more in line with ideas of trusteeship to give Africans precedence. Indians somehow fell between the cracks of British government policy – they were neither deemed a suitable official face for the imperial services of Kenya, nor regarded as the needy recipients of more official attention, as black Africans became from the mid-1920s.

The next chapter continues this theme of saving colonial faces by providing the book's one case study of non-cooperation. Here I take the example of the Zanzibar Maternity Association (ZMA), which was a local philanthropic organisation for the care of expectant mothers, started in 1918 and largely funded from charitable donations from Arab and Indian coffers. Actually the ZMA had originally been a British idea, and filled a conspicuous gap in the healthcare provision for women and children that the local Zanzibari Colonial Medical Service could not provide (it had no female MO), but the case study shows that the British were quick to distance themselves from the ZMA – even actively disparaging it – when their proposition to run it as an adjunct part of the colonial medical department was rejected by the local funders. This seems to be an example of the British rejecting cooperation when it was not precisely on the terms that they wanted. By revealing the limits to cooperation in this way, I expose some of the dominating preoccupations of the British Empire in the region: namely the desire to be seen to be fully in control.

Matthew Heaton's Chapter Six moves the scene to the interaction between the Colonial Medical Service in Nigeria and the private shipping company Elder Dempster, providing a rare example of the way the colonial authorities cooperated with private business as a means of repatriating back to colonial Nigeria persons deemed to be lunatics. Although the Colonial Office in London undertook much of the organisation of these repatriations, the local colonial medical departments had to confirm or deny each individual's home-coming. Furthermore, they created the preconditions for a patient's return by ensuring that the mental health infrastructure was in place for their care. This highlights the intricate tripartite negotiations that had to occur, both within and beyond the state, to facilitate the repatriation of those regarded as being insane. This three-way dialogue simultaneously reinforced fundamentally racist ideas of the periphery of Empire (i.e. the colonies) as the desired dumping ground for unfit African immigrants, rather than looking after them in European mental health institutions.

In Chapter Seven Shane Doyle adds another subtle strand to the analysis by arguing for the influence of non-medical research as a core determinant in the shaping of Colonial Medical Service policies and practice. Some of this research came from colonial departments outside the Colonial Medical Service, while others came from research organisations affiliated to, but not run by, the British state (such as the East African Institute for Social Research). Furthermore, to justify certain stances and interventions, Doyle shows how the medical department of Tanganyika regularly sought a broad variety of academic opinions, particularly from expert anthropologists, psychologists and ethnographers, to underpin its decisions and practices. By looking at the cases of the campaigns against sexually transmitted diseases in Buhaya, Tanganyika and malnutrition in Buganda, Uganda, Doyle is able to show how the Tanganyikan and Ugandan Colonial Medical Departments regularly looked outside their own immediate remits to bolster and secure their own socio-medical interventions.

[13]

Finally, in Chapter Eight we return to the relationship between the government medical service and the missions, this time with a specific eye to analysing the passage to post-colonial ideas of development. Mike Jennings uses Tanganyika as his case study and rounds off the volume by making the valuable and original point that colonial medicine was a progressively formalised joint endeavour between state and missionary healthcare providers. This, he points out, directly impacted on the subsequent development of the post-colonial voluntary sector in Tanzania after independence. Jennings looks particularly at the role of the Tanganyika Mission Council (established 1934) and the Medical Missionary Committee (established 1936) as formal representative bodies of the mission sector in Tanganyika, arguing that their establishment created the preconditions to make them a formal part of the Tanganyikan health sector. In an academic climate that always seems hungry to measure the 'impact' of studying history on the understanding of modern issues, Jennings's final conclusions are especially welcome. He persuasively argues that the modern 'encroachment of NGOs into the public space from the 1980s was, then, not something new, but a recasting of older forms of the delivery of public goods'. Missions should be seen, according to Jennings, as the originators of the voluntary sector and should be, along with state actors, part of our new histories of welfare and development.

Conclusion

The reach of the Colonial Medical Service went far beyond the state, with a significant number of members of the service collaborating, formally and informally, with a range of non-governmental groups, such as missionaries or those with commercial ties to Africa. Of course there were local differences – differences that sometimes existed within a single territory. Relations within the same government department with distinctive groups of non-state actors were likely to be differently adaptive to the particular circumstances of each engagement. For each example this book shows of government MOs working with non-government ones, a contrary example can no doubt be found elsewhere which does not convey such an easy harmony. It is not our intention to push an idealised image of a misunderstood Colonial Medical Service always keen to work with everyone, and with the health of the indigenous people as its only philanthropic intent. Far from it. Indeed, it is vital to grasp how cases of collaboration were nearly always ultimately coloured by colonial self-interest. At the end of the day, the Colonial Medical Service had to uphold government values, and when dissenters raised their voices too loudly they were likely to be kicked out.[40]

Similarly, irrespective of the fact that black and brown people also worked diligently within the medical department's framework, they were only exceptionally allowed to hold full ranking MO positions, even if their experience and medical qualifications were identical to, or even superior to, those held by their European colleagues. Yet, for all of its internal diversity, a strong sense of professional unity predominantly – if tenaciously – bound government officers together under the umbrella of their work for the British government. Yet, while cautioning against over-egging the pudding of a happy-go-lucky image of the comparatively free nature of colonial life, it is clear that the myth of unity that I wrote about in 2007 was too simplistic.

It might be useful to think of the Colonial Medical Service as one of the victims of the tyranny of the discipline of history itself. Certain parts of its history, because they were not palatable at the time, were simply not regularly spoken about and were recorded only indirectly (if at all) in the archive. National pressures – above all the importance of Empire building and, later, justifying it – subtly came to influence the way history has been written. Just as controversies were not good for the public face of Empire, neither were examples of collaboration. They somehow diluted the might of the imperial workforce and perhaps suggested that it was not as self-sufficient and dominant as the British government would have liked to present it as being.

Slowly we are getting to the heart of these understated, but nevertheless quite powerful, public relations exercises of the British colonial government. Recent scandals, such as the discovery of the thousands of hidden Colonial Office and Foreign Office files, should make us sit up and pay attention to the fact that colonial historians have only ever been fed a rather partial diet of historical facts.[41] The UK state archives are mostly open and accessible, but there are clearly still many things that historians do not know about, precisely because the Colonial Office and subsequent governments did not want us to know about them.[42] We are not exposing any great scandals within the pages that follow, but even gentle reassessments help us to reorientate our former understandings of past historical events. They remind us once again that history is always on the move. We will never be able to capture the full story, but each baby step brings us a little closer to understanding it a little better.

Notes

1 Anna Crozier, *Practising Colonial Medicine: The Colonial Medical Service in British East Africa*, London, I.B. Tauris, 2007
2 Anna Greenwood and Harshad Topiwala, *Indian Doctors in Kenya: The Forgotten Story, 1895–1940*, forthcoming, London, Palgrave Macmillan, 2015
3 Most recently, Ryan Johnson and Amna Khalid (eds.), *Public Health in the British*

Empire: Intermediaries, Subordinates, and the Practice of Public Health, New York and London, Routledge, 2012

4   Indeed the social background and academic qualifications of many Colonial Medical Service employees were often modest compared to those of their contemporaries in the Colonial Administrative Service. See Crozier, *Practising Colonial Medicine*, p. 106

5   The Foreign Office managed the African colonies until the early 1900s, at which point most African territories (except Sudan and Egypt) moved under the Colonial Office. The India Office managed the area now covered by the modern territories of India, Pakistan, Myanmar and Bangladesh.

6   For a full history see: Cosmo Parkinson, *The Colonial Office from Within, 1909–1945*, London, Faber and Faber Ltd., 1947; Charles Jeffries, *Partners for Progress: The Men and Women of the Colonial Service*, London, George G. Harrap, 1949; Anthony Kirk-Greene, *On Crown Service: A History of HM Colonial and Overseas Civil Services, 1837–1997*, London, I.B. Tauris, 1999; John Smith (ed.), *Administering Empire: The British Colonial Service in Retrospect*, London, University of London Press, 1999; Anthony Kirk-Greene, *Britain's Imperial Administrators, 1858–1966*, London, Macmillan, 2000

7   Kirk-Greene, *On Crown Service*, p. 11

8   Colonial Office, 'Report of the Committee Chaired by Sir Warren Fisher', *The System of Appointment in the Colonial Office and the Colonial Services*, London, HMSO, 1930

9   Charles Jeffries, *The Colonial Empire and its Civil Service*, Cambridge, Cambridge University Press, 1938, pp. 16–17; Colonial Office, Cmd. 939 *Report of the Departmental Committee Appointed by the Secretary of State for the Colonies to Enquire into the Colonial Medical Services*, London, HMSO, 1920, p. 6

10   Anthony Kirk-Greene, *A Biographical Dictionary of the British Colonial Service, 1939–1966*, London, H. Zell, 1991, pp. v–vi

11   Kirk-Greene, *On Crown Service*, p. 16

12   Although the position was not formally ratified as being Chief Medical Advisor to the Colonial Office until 1926, Manson held the position *de facto* from 1897.

13   H.J.O.D. Burke-Gaffney, 'The History of Medicine in the African Countries', *Medical History*, 12, 1968, pp. 31–41, pp. 33–4; Anon, 'Instruction in Tropical Diseases', *British Medical Journal*, i, 1895, p. 771

14   See H.C. Squires, *The Sudan Medical Service: An Experiment in Social Medicine*, London, William Heinemann, 1958, p. 14; Heather Bell, *Frontiers of Medicine in the Anglo-Egyptian Sudan, 1899–1940*, Oxford, Clarendon Press 1999, pp. 39–40

15   Mark Harrison, *Public Health in British India: Anglo-Indian Preventative Medicine 1859–1914*, Cambridge, Cambridge University Press, 1994, pp. 27–35

16   This is the 1893 case of West African John Farrell Easmon. Although once the WAMS was amalgamated in 1902 an explicitly racist entry policy was instituted. Ryan Johnson, '"An All-White Institution": Defending Private Practice and the Formation of the West African Medical Staff', *Medical History*, 54, 2010, pp. 237–54, p. 238

17   Ranajit Guha, 'The Small Voices of History', in Shahid Amin and Dipesh Chakrabarty (eds.), *Subaltern Studies: Writings on South Asian History and Society*, Vol. IX, Oxford, Oxford University Press, 1988, pp. 1–12

18   Greenwood and Topiwala, *Indian Doctors*

19   Crozier, *Practising Colonial Medicine*, pp. 19–31

20   For a detailed explanation of this see James Anthony Mangan, *'Benefits Bestowed'? Education and British Imperialism*, Manchester, Manchester University Press, 1988

21   The National Archives, UK (TNA) CO/877/1/37811 Ralph Furse, 'Proposal for Holding the Tropical African Services Course at Oxford and Cambridge', 1 April 1920

22   RHL (Rhodes House Library, Oxford) Mss.Brit.Emp.s.415 Furse Papers, Memorandum Furse to Lord Milner 18 June 1918.

23 Colonial Office, *Miscellaneous No. 99: Colonial Medical Appointments*, London, The Colonial Office, 1921; Colonial Office, *Miscellaneous No. 488: The Colonial Service, General Conditions of Employment*, London, The Colonial Office, 1939

24 Crozier, *Practising Colonial Medicine*, p. 50

25 For example: RHL MSS.Afr.s.1872/82 James Kellock Hunter 'Detailed Memorandum on Experiences in the Colonial Medical Service in Uganda, 1939–58' [n.d., c.1983], p. 19

26 Colin Baker, 'The Government Medical Service in Malawi: an Administrative History, 1891–1974', *Medical History*, 20, 1976, pp. 450–65; A. Bayoumi, *The History of the Sudan Health Services*, Nairobi, Kenya Literature Bureau, 1979; Ann Beck, *A History of the British Medical Administration of East Africa: 1900–1950*, Cambridge, MA, Harvard University Press, 1970; Mary Bull, *The Medical Services of Uganda 1954–5*, Report 20, Oxford Development Records Project, Rhodes House Library, Oxford, [n.d., c.198?]; Mary Bull, *The Medical Services of Tanganyika 1955*, Report 21, Oxford Development Records Project, Rhodes House Library, Oxford, [n.d., c.198?]; David F. Clyde, *History of the Medical Services of Tanganyika*, Dar es Salaam, Government Press, 1962; W.D. Foster, 'Robert Moffat and the Beginnings of the Government Medical Service in Uganda', *Medical History*, 13, 1969, pp. 237–50; W.D. Foster, *The Early History of Scientific Medicine in Uganda*, Nairobi, East Africa Literature Bureau, 1970; Michael Gelfand, *A Service to the Sick: A History of the Health Services for Africans in Southern Rhodesia, 1890–1953*, Gweru, Mambo Press, 1976; Judith N. Lasker, 'The Role of Health Services in Colonial Rule: the Case of the Ivory Coast', *Culture, Medicine and Psychiatry*, 1, 1977, pp. 277–97; Ralph Schram, *A History of the Nigerian Health Services*, Ibadan, Ibadan University Press, 1971; Squires, *Sudan Medical Service*

27 Crozier, *Practising Colonial Medicine*; Johnson, '"An All-White Institution"'; Ryan Johnson, 'The West African Medical Staff and the Administration of Imperial Tropical Medicine, 1902–14', *The Journal of Imperial and Commonwealth History*, 38, 3, 2010, pp. 419–39

28 Some of these old grand narratives include: Michael Gelfand, *Tropical Victory: An Account of the Influence of Medicine on the History of Southern Rhodesia, 1900–1923*, Cape Town, Juta, 1953; Aldo Castellani, *Microbes, Men and Monarchs: A Doctor's Life in Many Lands*, London, Gollancz, 1960; Schram, *History of the Nigerian Health Services*; J.J. McKelvey Jr, *Man Against Tsetse: Struggle for Africa*, London, Cornell University Press, 1973; Gelfand, *A Service to the Sick*

29 Daniel R. Headrick, *The Tools of Empire: Technology and European Imperialism in the Nineteenth Century*, Oxford, Oxford University Press, 1981 (see also Roy Macleod and Milton Lewis (eds.), *Disease Medicine and Empire*, London, Routledge, 1988)

30 Randall Packard, *White Plague, Black Labor: Tuberculosis and the Political Economy of Health and Disease in South Africa*, Berkeley, University of California Press, 1989; Megan Vaughan, *Curing Their Ills: Colonial Power and African Illness*, Cambridge, Polity Press, 1991; John Farley, *Bilharzia: A History of Imperial Tropical Medicine*, Cambridge, Cambridge University Press, 2008 [first published 1991]; Maryinez Lyons, *The Colonial Disease: A Social History of Sleeping Sickness in Northern Zaire 1900–1940*, Cambridge, Cambridge University Press, 2002 [first published, 1992]; Harrison, *Public Health in British India*; Sanjoy Bhattacharya, *Expunging Variola: The Control and Eradication of Smallpox in India, 1947–1977*, New Delhi and London, Orient Longman India and Sangam Books, 2006

31 David Arnold, *Colonizing the Body: State Medicine and Epidemic Disease in Nineteenth Century India*, Berkeley, University of California Press, 1993

32 David Hardiman and Projit Mukharji (eds.), *Medical Marginality in South Asia: Situating Subaltern Therapeutics*, London, Routledge, 2012

33 John Iliffe, *East African Doctors: A History of the Modern Profession*, Cambridge, Cambridge University Press, 1998; Anne Digby and Helen Sweet, 'The Nurse as Culture Broker in Twentieth Century South Africa', in Waltraud Ernst (ed.), *Plural Medicine, Tradition and Modernity*, London, Routledge, 2002, pp. 113–29; Philip D.

Morgan and Sean Hawkins (eds.), *Black Experience and the Empire*, Oxford, Oxford University Press, 2004; Benjamin N. Lawrance, Emily Lynn Osborn and Richard L Roberts (eds.), *Intermediaries, Interpreters, and Clerks: African Employees in the Making of Colonial Africa*, Madison, University of Wisconsin Press, 2006; Anne-Marie Rafferty, 'The Rise and Demise of the Colonial Nursing Service: British Nurses in the Colonies, 1896–1966', *Nursing History Review*, 15, 2007, pp. 147–54; Johnson and Khalid (eds.), *Public Health in the British Empire*

34 Waltraud Ernst (ed.), *Plural Medicine, Tradition and Modernity*, London, Routledge, 2002; Pratik Chakrabarti, *Western Science in Modern India: Metropolitan Methods, Colonial Practices*, Delhi, Permanent Black, 2004; Sanjoy Bhattacharya, Mark Harrison and Michael Worboys (eds.), *Fractured States: Smallpox, Public Health and Vaccination Policy in British India, 1800–1947*, New Delhi, Orient Longman and Sangam Books, 2005; Anne Digby, *Diversity and Division in Medicine: Healthcare in South Africa from the 1800s*, Oxford, Peter Lang, 2006; Guy Attewell, *Refiguring Unani Tibb: Plural Healing in Late Colonial India*, New Delhi, Orient Longman, 2007; Biswamoy Pati and Mark Harrison (eds.), *The Social History of Health and Medicine in Colonial India*, London and New York, Routledge, 2009; Hormoz Ebrahimnejad (ed.), *The Development of Modern Medicine in Non-Western Countries: Historical Perspectives*, London and New York, Routledge, 2009

35 Dane Kennedy and Durba Ghosh (eds.), *Decentring Empire: Britain, India, and the Transcolonial World*, New Delhi, Longman Orient Press, 2006; Kevin Grant, Philippa Levine and Frank Trentmann (eds.), *Beyond Sovereignty, 1880–1950: Britain, Empire and Transnationalism*, London, Palgrave, 2007; Pratik Chakrabarti, *Medicine and Empire, 1600–1960*, London, Palgrave Macmillan, 2013

36 Alan Lester, *Imperial Networks: Creating Identities in Nineteenth-Century South Africa and Britain*, London, Routledge, 2001; Alan Lester, 'Imperial Circuits and Networks: Geographies of the British Empire', *History Compass*, 4, 2006, pp. 124–41; Zoe Laidlaw, *Colonial Connections 1815–45: Patronage, the Information Revolution and Colonial Government*, Manchester, Manchester University Press, 2005; Simon J. Potter, 'Webs, Networks and Systems: Globalization and the Mass Media in the Nineteenth- and Twentieth-Century British Empire', *Journal of British Studies*, 46, 2007, pp. 621–46; Brett M Bennett and Joseph M. Hodge (eds.), *Science and Empire: Knowledge and Networks of Science Across the British Empire, 1800–1970*, Basingstoke, Palgrave Macmillan, 2011; Deborah J. Neill, *Networks in Tropical Medicine: Internationalism, Colonialism, and the Rise of a Medical Specialty, 1890–1930*, Stanford, Stanford University Press, 2012

37 David Hardiman (ed.), *Healing Bodies, Saving Souls: Medical Missions in Asia and Africa*, Amsterdam and New York, Rodopi, 2006; David Hardiman, *Missionaries and Their Medicine: A Christian Modernity for Tribal India*, Manchester and New York, Manchester University Press, 2008; Charles Good, *The Steamer Parish: The Rise and Fall of Missionary Medicine in an African Frontier*, London, University of Chicago Press, 2004; Markku Hokkanen, *Medicine and Scottish Missionaries in the Northern Malawi Region: Quests for Health in a Colonial Society*, Lewiston, The Edwin Mellen Press, 2007

38 James Midgley and David Piachaud (eds.), *Colonialism and Welfare: Social Policy and the British Imperial Legacy*, London, Edward Elgar Publishing, 2012

39 Sanjoy Bhattacharya with Sharon Messenger, *The Global Eradication of Smallpox*, Hyderabad, Orient Black Swan, 2010

40 The use of the acceptable diagnosis of tropical neurasthenia as a pretext to do this can be seen in Anna Crozier, 'What was Tropical about Tropical Neurasthenia? The Utility of the Diagnosis in the Management of Empire', *Journal for the History of Medicine and Allied Sciences*, 64, 4, 2009, pp. 518–48

41 Ian Cobain, 'Foreign Office Hoarding 1m Historic Files in Secret Archive', *Guardian*, 18 October 2013; Ian Cobain, 'Revealed: the Bonfire of Papers at the End of Empire', *Guardian*, 29 November 2013

42 A big revelation was David Anderson, *Histories of the Hanged: The Dirty War in Kenya and the End of Empire*, London, Weidenfeld and Nicolson, 2005

CHAPTER TWO

Crossing the divide: medical missionaries and government service in Uganda, 1897–1940

Yolana Pringle

One of the distinctive features of Western medical practice in early colonial Uganda was the high level of collaboration between mission doctors and the Colonial Medical Service.[1] In the period before 1940, a number of Church Missionary Society (CMS) doctors negotiated dual roles as missionaries and colonial medical officers. An even greater number participated in and managed government health campaigns, or were engaged unofficially by the administration in an advisory capacity. The reasons for collaboration were diverse: some wished to extend the reach of missionary work, some to advance professionally, while others were determined to boost what they felt to be meagre missionary stipends. By undertaking this work, the mission doctors went beyond filling a gap in state provision: they contributed specialist knowledge, language skills, equipment and personnel that shaped the practice of the Colonial Medical Service in Uganda as much as they supplemented it. However, the relationship was never clearly defined. Stemming in part from the inability to draw an absolute line between 'missionary' and 'government' medical work, missionaries and colonial administrators reacted to local circumstances, formulating guidelines in a largely *ad hoc* manner.

Historians of medicine have explored the numerous ways in which missionaries and government officials came together in Uganda.[2] While these historians have not always focused on the relationship between medical missionaries and the Colonial Medical Service per se, their work has indicated that the boundary between the two was often fluid. Carol Summers, for example, has shown how the establishment of the Maternity Training School in Uganda represented 'a joint venture between the state and its missionary subcontractor, two groups with different agendas but overlapping interests'.[3] John Iliffe has set out the ways in which medical education schemes in East Africa, and Uganda in particular, developed directly from the early efforts of medical missionaries to train tribal dressers and African medical assistants.[4] Anna Greenwood has noted how the divide between missionaries and government officials in East Africa was not always clear cut.[5] Some joined the Colonial Medical Service having been rejected by a missionary society, whereas others felt a calling to join the Church in their retirement. And more recently Kathleen Vongsathorn, looking specifically at the theme of cooperation, has argued that missionaries and government officials put aside their differences to engineer model leprosy settlements for the relief of suffering.[6]

In Uganda, the contribution of missionaries to the development of government medical services has not been downplayed or marginalised to the extent it has been elsewhere in colonial Africa.[7] This is due in part to early historians of medicine in Uganda, admittedly some themselves missionaries, who have stressed the debt of the colonial administration to the pioneer medical work and research started by Albert Ruskin Cook.[8] It also stems from the extensive collection of records deposited by the CMS in archives at the University of Birmingham (UK), the Wellcome Library (UK), Uganda Christian University (Mukono, Uganda), and the Albert Cook Library (Makerere University, Uganda). This has resulted in a bias in the historical literature towards CMS activities, and specifically those initiated by Albert Cook. Roman Catholic missionaries were also engaged in a number of medical projects, including leprosy and maternal health, but the difficulties historians have experienced in accessing archival material has resulted in little critical analysis of their work.[9] It is beyond the remit of this chapter to redress this bias, but the interest of historians of missionary medicine – Catholic or Protestant – in medical 'projects', such as the training of doctors, maternal health, venereal diseases, or leprosy, has led to a related skew in the historical literature, the focus of which is the starting point for this piece. CMS medical missionaries collaborated with the colonial government on a number of campaigns, but this does not necessarily mean that they came together only when their interests converged. What has yet to be explored in a medical context in Uganda is the multiple ways that missionaries and government officials came together on a more mundane, day-to-day basis, assisting and offering advice even when it was not necessarily in the mission's or government's best interests. These activities brought together mission and government doctors as professional colleagues and 'experts', and in turn shaped what both 'missionary medicine' and 'colonial medicine' could offer to patients.

This chapter examines the practicalities of the relationship between medical missionaries and colonial administrators in the period before 1940, focusing primarily on CMS mission doctors. It starts by considering the everyday dealings between mission doctors and the colonial government at the CMS Mengo Hospital, founded by Albert Cook in 1897.[10] It then turns to CMS hospitals elsewhere in Uganda, looking at how the Colonial Medical Service sought in the 1920s to formalise their relationship with individual mission doctors. This is followed by a section that investigates how increased government funding for individual projects, campaigns, and hospitals eventually shifted the nature of colonial medicine in Uganda, and with it the relationship between missionaries and the colonial government. The chapter ends by briefly considering the patients themselves. Indeed, it is important to remember that while the sharing of specialist knowledge, equipment, and personnel assisted in extending the reach of Western medicine, both mission and government doctors remained on the periphery of a much broader therapeutic landscape in Uganda.

Mengo Hospital, 1897–1920

In the early years of colonial rule, the relationship between mission and government doctors was determined largely by practical circumstances. Government medical provision, as Robert Moffat, Principal Medical Officer (PMO), complained in 1903, was almost non-existent: there were no native hospitals that could 'be dignified by the name', and those that did consisted 'generally of small temporary sheds or huts in which a sick man can be sheltered'.[11] For Moffat, the lack of facilities not only affected staff morale, but had serious implications for the scientific study of disease:

> In hospital cases can be carefully watched and studied and in this way far more information can be obtained in regard to diseases which may be prevalent or peculiar to the country than can be got in an out patient consulting room. For this reason the returns and records of the work done by Government Medical Officers are for the most part valueless. The work done by the Mission Doctors at their hospital in Namirembe is in contrast and they are often enabled to record the presence or prevalence of diseases even the names of which never find a place in my reports.[12]

The importance of Mengo Hospital, Namirembe, in identifying disease had already been demonstrated. In 1901, brothers and fellow mission doctors Albert and Jack Cook had notified the colonial government and the medical community in Britain of concerns over the growing number of sleeping sickness cases arriving at their hospital, sparking international interest in a disease that was to devastate local communities on the shores of Lake Victoria.[13] The role assumed by mission doctors at Mengo Hospital, and the manner in which they informed

[21]

and advised the Colonial Medical Service, was to shape government medical practice in Uganda for the next thirty years.

The ability of mission doctors to communicate with patients in a number of local languages, combined with their attention to record keeping, meant that the doctors at Mengo Hospital were looked upon as having exceptional insight into local health and disease conditions. Of particular interest were Mengo Hospital's records on sleeping sickness, plague, blackwater fever, venereal diseases, and enteric fever, which were repeatedly searched for information on the frequency, etiological signs, and geographical distribution of disease.[14] In August 1916, C.J. Baker, Medical Sanitary Officer, even went so far as to apologise for his repeated requests for information from the mission hospital, but stressed the effect they could have on government policy – if any local cases of enteric fever could be found in Mengo Hospital's collection of patient case notes, it 'would strengthen a plea for a piped water supply for the town'.[15]

Stemming in part from their location on the outskirts of Kampala Township and their extended presence in the region, the mission doctors at Mengo Hospital were considered to have 'strong ideas' on government policy affecting Kampala, and were frequently consulted by senior officials on an unofficial basis.[16] Advice was sought on aspects of medical practice, hygiene, sanitation, and town planning, demonstrating both the influence of mission doctors within government circles and how the reach of missionary medicine extended beyond their own curative services. Such was the volume of correspondence, Albert Cook noted in 1919, coming from 'all over both Protectorates, sometimes entailing 20 letters a day, all the Administrative work of a large Hospital, keeping in touch with Govt Officials, looking after Affiliated Dispensaries, needful Indents, as well as the purely Professional side of the work', that he felt exhausted and in desperate need of a secretary.[17]

Certainly, in addition to their own patients, the doctors at Mengo Hospital advised on difficult cases by post and accepted patients referred by colonial medical officers from across Uganda. While these patients were predominantly European, a number of African and Indian cases were also sent for operations and specialist treatment.[18] Between 1912 and 1938, Mengo Hospital housed the only X-ray equipment in Uganda, and patients requiring X-rays were sent to the hospital by government officials from around the country.[19] In 1915, Jack Cook also received two convicted murderers – one for a broken arm and the other for observations on his mental state.[20] In this instance, as in other cases, no restrictions were placed on the spiritual side of the mission doctors' work. While additional fees may have come from the colonial government, patients were admitted on the same basis as other patients, and were obliged to attend daily prayers and ward services.

Over time, this professional relationship was strengthened by the formation of an intellectual community in Kampala. From its establishment in 1913, mission and government doctors met regularly at meetings of the Uganda branch of the British Medical Association (BMA) and while on furlough in London.[21] In addition to being a powerful lobbying voice for the Colonial Medical Service, the local branch of the BMA also provided a forum through which doctors could come together as medical colleagues and professional experts. At the first Presidential Address, for example, held at Mengo Hospital in December 1913, Albert Cook presented a paper on obstetrics in Uganda, to which both colonial medical officers and other mission doctors offered their opinions on clinical cases and patient fees.[22] Mission and government doctors also corresponded privately on interesting cases and particular aspects of research, offering feedback on papers for submission to scientific journals.[23]

Mission and government hospitals both suffered from a lack of specialist facilities and staff, necessitating cooperation on the level of general medical practice and research. Of course, much of this assistance was rooted in financial concerns, but it was also reflective of a more general collaboration between mission and government doctors that was not regarded as exceptional. Indeed, before the 1920s, the close working relationship between the doctors at Mengo Hospital and the Colonial Medical Service caused little controversy; while the anti-venereal, motherhood, and education campaigns were accompanied by negotiations on the boundaries between mission and government responsibilities and the place of religion, there were no clear guidelines on the appropriateness of their other professional activities. In their published writings, the mission doctors also presented a number of aspects of their day-to-day collaboration with the Colonial Medical Service as examples of the mission's importance, both for Britain and for the Empire as a whole. This was most overt during the First World War, when Mengo Hospital was used as a government base hospital for the war in East Africa. Commenting on the policy of the CMS with regard to war service, J.H. Cook noted in *Mercy and Truth*, the medical journal of the CMS, how 'on the one hand, missionary duties have not prevented our missionaries and doctors from offering their services to their country in connexion with the war; and, on the other hand, war service has not curtailed, but has greatly increased, the scope and opportunities of their missionary labours'.[24]

Much of the discretion held by the mission doctors in their daily activities stemmed from the fact that the 'missionary' element of medical mission work was never well defined. On the one hand, medical missions were presented as a way of reaching potential converts – natives would be 'dazzled' by Western medicine and become more receptive to the Christian message as a result.[25] On the other, even more 'secular' medical activities, such as research, could benefit the mission by enabling the hospital to offer the latest therapeutic techniques and so cater for an increasingly demanding patient population.[26] In their general medical practice, at least, the doctors at Mengo Hospital found it impossible to draw a line between the two; requests for advice and consultations were unexceptional, and even to be expected, given their long presence in the region. By tacitly fulfilling these roles, however, the mission doctors were shaping the activities of the Colonial Medical Service, and involving themselves in both policy and practice.

Half-time workers

If the everyday relationship between medical missionaries and the Colonial Medical Service had been relatively unproblematic, it was to emerge as an area requiring definition and regulation in the early 1920s. Faced with the need to increase the size and scope of government medical provision at minimal cost, administrators started to attempt to harness missionary manpower through formal arrangements.[27] In Western Province, encompassing Ankole, Toro, and Kigezi Districts, this involved the creation of a new type of post, that of the 'half-time' District Medical Officer (DMO). Between 1921 and 1928, at least four CMS medical missionaries posted to Toro and Kigezi – Alfred Schofield, Ernest Cook, Algie Stanley Smith, and Leonard Sharp – took on dual roles as missionaries and colonial medical officers.[28] For the mission doctors, this arrangement allowed them access to additional facilities and equipment, as well as providing them with the opportunity to gain extra money for the mission. For the government, the formal co-opting of mission doctors into the Colonial Medical Service allowed for the façade that government medical provision was expanding at an impressively cost-effective rate.

The first mission doctor to be approached in this way was Ashton Bond, founder and head of the CMS Kabarole Hospital, Fort Portal. Bond had been the sole Western medical practitioner in Toro District since 1903, and had long undertaken work for the colonial government on an unofficial basis.[29] As early as 1911, Bond had expanded his ordinary hospital work to include visits to native and government prisons, provided colonial administrators with statistics, toured the sub-counties, and provided district and provincial administrators with advice.[30] By 1920, Bond also had sole responsibility for the treatment of European government officials and the official medical management of epidemics, which in 1919–20 involved a serious outbreak of cerebro-spinal meningitis.[31] While the work did not go unappreciated by the Colonial Medical Service, it was not paid, and no formal arrangement had been made. Indeed, Bond had long seen this work as part of his 'daily routine': it neither interfered with his CMS work, nor could be easily separated from it.[32]

Early in 1920, Bond approached the PMO, independently of the CMS, and asked to receive part of the fees paid by the government for his medical work. Recognising the Uganda government's inability to send a colonial medical officer to Toro, while feeling increasingly obliged to expand government medical services, the PMO agreed.[33] The CMS authorities in London balked at the proposed arrangement: missionaries were not to make personal agreements with the government, and they were certainly not to receive any payment in addition to their missionary stipend. In a letter to Bond in May 1920, George Manley, CMS Secretary with primary responsibility for East Africa, noted that: 'We think you would act quite rightly if you were to point out to the government that you are already fully employed with your CMS work, that you had gone out on the understanding that you would give your whole time to that [and] that you must therefore decline to undertake any work on behalf of the government'.[34] Manley was well aware that the distinction between missionary and strictly secular medical work could be blurred, but the prospect of a formal agreement and personal remuneration for Bond had forced him to set out the limits.[35]

It was these concerns about mission authority and money, rather than the nature of the work, which were repeated when the issue of Bond's appointment resurfaced in October 1920. Keenly aware that the Colonial Medical Service still had no presence in Toro District, the PMO offered Bond an allowance as a half-time medical officer. Without consulting the CMS, Bond accepted. Enraged at what he saw as the hypocrisy of the CMS when it came to receiving money from the government, Bond pointed out that CMS missionaries who took Sunday services for government officials received fees and a small travel allowance: 'There is nothing I consider (and the government agree) different in principle to the clergy receiving an allowance for taking a service for government officials, and others, on a Sunday, and my receiving an allowance for medical and official work which I do for them on weekdays.'[36] In Bond's opinion, the extra payment would not only be fair, but necessary in a country like Uganda, where the cost of living was so high.[37] Unsurprisingly, the CMS again ordered Bond to decline any formal agreement. Pointing out that Bond was not 'at

Liberty' to negotiate with the government, the local Secretary of the Uganda Mission, based at Namirembe, stressed that if Bond felt 'that he would be happier under Government', he could give six months' notice of his intention to resign.[38]

The situation was somewhat different when Sharp was appointed as half-time DMO for Kigezi, with the sanction of the CMS in London and Namirembe, in the following year. Mission medical work in Kigezi had been approved only on the basis that the bulk of the costs for the first four years would be from extra-mission sources.[39] Permission had been granted to seek a large government grant for the mission, but while no large grant was forthcoming, the colonial administration was willing to subsidise work in the form of making Sharp a half-time Medical Officer. This suited both parties: the CMS would have a small income for its mission as well as immediate use of hospital buildings at Kabale, and government medical work would officially be extended into Kigezi.[40]

Clearly unaware of the purpose of the funds in the Kigezi case, Bond took issue with the new agreement. Highlighting what he saw as inconsistency between CMS rules and practice, he asked how other extra-mission activities – including private medical practice and land-ownership – were not proscribed.[41] Adding to this the low stipends granted to missionaries in the field, Bond stressed how he could not 'accept ... [the] ... view that a missionary has sold himself body + soul to the society, + that they may not accept any remuneration except what they receive from the society'.[42] This tension between Bond and his superiors mirrors wider debates that occurred within the Colonial Medical Service over whether government medical officers should be allowed to engage in private practice.[43] Government service was associated with loyalty not just to colleagues, but also to the British government. Thus, while the CMS allowed its doctors to participate in private practice, it was particularly sensitive about arrangements with the government that might lessen its control over mission workers.

Sharp was unable to ignore his commitment to missionary work while attached to the Colonial Medical Service in Kigezi. Some areas of work could be clearly delineated financially, of course: the administration of government dispensaries, for example, comprised a major part of Sharp's duties as DMO.[44] But much was also left to Sharp's discretion, including the investigation of outbreaks of disease, permission to delegate duties to his missionary colleague, Stanley Smith, and his evangelical work.[45] Having been reported to have compelled patients at the government-owned Kabale Hospital buildings to attend religious services, for example, Sharp noted that: 'I am using these buildings as though they were Missions premises and ... regular services have been started for the patients ... In this connection I must mention that it is one of the first rules of C.M.S. Mission Hospitals that all patients should attend the service.'[46] Sharp had earlier criticised medical practice at Mengo Hospital for 'becoming more + more philanthropic in contradistinction to missionary in character', and did not intend his own work to follow the same pattern.[47] As the Provincial Commissioner (PC), Western Province, conceded in 1922:

> It would not appear possible for Dr. Sharp to draw any dividing line between his Government and Missionary work and as long as the Government employs a half time District Medical Officer, I think it must allow him full discretion over his work and leave to you any steps you may think fit to lay down as regards the supervision of his work on tour. I would therefore recommend the withdrawal of the words 'when travelling solely on Government duty' and substitute 'while carrying out Government work'. In this way the present difficulty raised by the District Commissioner will be avoided, and it will be left to Dr. Sharp to carry out his Government duties on tour along with his Missionary work.[48]

A similar amount of discretion was granted to the CMS mission doctors who were employed as part-time DMOs in Toro District. Following Bond's abortive attempt to seek payment for his unofficial government work, Ernest Cook and Schofield were granted permission to make formal arrangements with the Colonial Medical Service, with money going to the mission.[49] Recalling the reasons behind the arrangement ten years later, Schofield noted how, despite the feeling that government service would be 'a hindrance to my missionary work', the extra money it allowed the mission was irresistible. He attributed similar financial concerns to the colonial administration:

> Every Government Doctor cost the Government £1,600 to £1,750 per year, apart altogether from the cost of the work he did. This figure was simply what it cost to keep a Doctor, for instance, at Toro – his house allowance, and all other allowances, part of a wife's passage, his own passage and cost of relief during holiday, in other words, the same sort of figures we have to work on in the Mission are £600 (average). But in addition to this sum there had also to be taken into account the material, drugs, maintenance of buildings, wages of his assistants and everything else and that estimate came to between £4,000 and £5,000 per Doctor per year. Of course that meant a lot of medical work and a lot of people seen and a lot of people treated, but (and this was the argument used to me by the P.M.O. at the time) that if they gave us a *quarter* of that amount of money we would be able to do the same amount of work.[50]

Despite mutual financial advantages, however, the part-time nature of the work was increasingly deemed to be inadequate. Not only were the mission doctors prohibited from evangelising while undertaking duties for the government, however ill-defined, but medical work on both sides was suffering.[51] In March 1923 it was noted that patients in Kigezi were shuttled between the government and CMS hospital, with the Sub-Assistant Surgeon, under Sharp, dealing 'with the local native sick, police, porters etc. and ... [keeping] ... the hospital records and care of stores; cases requiring special treatment being sent to the C.M.S. Hospital'.[52] In Toro, too, the PC, Western Province, noted in March 1925 that the 'District Medical Officer must of necessity expend nearly all his time at his Hospital at Kabarole and has consequently little chance of supervising the work of the County Dispensaries'.[53] 'Likewise', he continued, the DMO 'cannot do any touring should any infectious disease break out, he is practically tied to his Headquarters.'[54] Adding that this was not a criticism of the work done by the mission hospital, the PC finally stressed that:

> From the Mission point of view I doubt either whether the present arrangement can be considered entirely suitable as the Government duties to be performed must to a considerable extent prevent the Mission Doctor from carrying out the full Mission duties which he would otherwise perform, nor would the £300 received by the Mission be in this respect commensurate.[55]

Ultimately, the arrangement was criticised primarily for resulting in the underdevelopment of government medical provision in Western Province. With the existence of mission hospitals at Kabale and Fort Portal, coupled with a policy that privileged development in Buganda and Eastern Province, Western Province had been ignored.[56] By 1925, the only permanent government hospital building in Western Province was at Mbarara, Ankole District. A small temporary building was in use at Kabale, while at Toro the government relied completely on the CMS hospital.[57] These facts were an increasing embarrassment for the Colonial Medical Service, and in 1925 a full-time DMO was appointed to Toro District. The half-time arrangements held at Kigezi for longer, in part because the District was much smaller, but in 1929 that arrangement, too, was terminated.[58]

Mengo Hospital, 1921–40

The presence of colonial medical officers at Kampala and Entebbe meant that the doctors at Mengo Hospital were not called on as 'half-time' workers in the way they were elsewhere in Uganda. But attempts to extend government medical work did not go unnoticed by those working at Namirembe, who recognised the threat this posed to their own activities. At a meeting in 1923, medical and non-medical missionaries noted that while the government appeared anxious to work with the CMS, experience had shown that 'where Government Centres were astablished [sic] the C.M.S. work would be extinguished'.[59] The efforts of the doctors at Mengo Hospital to train African medical assistants were a particularly sore example of this, with government funding having recently been redirected to its own Medical School at Mulago Hospital.[60] The mission doctors who trained them had intended African medical assistants to take on basic clinical duties and to go out into 'untouched' regions to fight 'heathenism' and the traditional 'medicine-man'.[61] In practice, the relationship between African doctors and Western medicine was more ambiguous, and they would struggle with the CMS and the Colonial Medical Service over their status, duties, and right to private practice for the next thirty years.[62]

The desire to maintain missionary influence in colonial medical practice was a key reason for increased collaboration between mission and government doctors at Mengo Hospital, most notably through projects and campaigns, but also through individual arrangements. Following the failure of the CMS to secure government funding for a hygiene and education campaign, the Colonial Medical Service requested the 'loan or transfer' of Ernest Cook for medical education work at Mulago Medical School from 1925. Keen to have someone on the inside of the new school, and aware that internal disagreements between staff at Mengo Hospital meant there was no obvious place for Ernest Cook in its established medical mission work, the CMS agreed. But discussions over his secondment, and Ernest Cook's eventual decision to remain in the Colonial Medical Service permanently, raised similar issues over understandings of the 'missionary' element of medical missionary practice in Uganda as it had done elsewhere.

Writing to Ernest Cook in 1928, shortly before he decided to leave the CMS, Albert Cook noted that:

> You have been brought up to the cross roads once more & must decide one way or the other which road to take, & the choice this time seems to be final. On the one hand there is continuing in Govt service, receiving as you told me £800 a year at present, and an increasing scale of pay. You are doing there really useful work, valued by them & by the Baganda alike, and are showing a really fine Christian witness. On the other hand you do not feel the atmosphere from a missionary point of view is congenial. You … have no freedom to preach Christ to the patients in the Hospital, your Christian work, apart from the very powerful effect of example, must be out of hours & indirect.[63]

[29]

At the heart of it, while Albert Cook maintained that medical work could serve a Christian purpose anywhere, it was the attachment to a society that made a missionary: 'I sincerely believe that the Return of our Lord is very imminent, & may take place at any moment. Would you not like Him to find you in C.M.S. ranks? Even though you can do, very real work for Him at Mulago?'[64] Taking a rather different view of the role of the missionary, Ernest Cook defended his position, telling his uncle that:

> Apparently you are taking it for granted that the will of God for us lies necessarily in the C.M.S. and that we are seeking our own way if we do not go back.... I try to work as in His sight always, and our location here is not of our seeking – why should I be ashamed of it when He comes?[65]

When Ernest Cook finally decided to remain in the Colonial Medical Service, he did so primarily for financial reasons, and in so doing joined a number of other medical practitioners who both engaged with Christian ideals and sought a higher-paying alternative to missionary life.[66]

Among the doctors at Mengo Hospital, the financial pressures arising from the post-war reduction in missionary subscriptions, coupled with increased competition from government hospitals, meant that even those remaining in missionary service felt it necessary to focus on the more 'secular' aspects of medical work.[67] This they did with increasing autonomy, using the hospital's status as self-supporting to disregard the authority of the local missionary governing board at Namirembe.[68] Most prominent among these activities were medical consultations, which had multiplied with the opening of new government hospitals in the early 1920s. Mengo Hospital continued to house the only X-ray equipment in Uganda until 1938, and at least one of its doctors, Robert Stones, was a noted ophthalmologist.[69]

The professional collaboration between mission and government doctors was not one way. Indeed, the doctors at Mengo Hospital were reliant on the laboratory at Mulago Hospital for Wasserman reaction tests, the CMS being unable to afford the equipment or the time to conduct its own tests for syphilis.[70] There was also an increasing presence of colonial medical officers in the Uganda branch of the BMA, which held its first meeting at Mulago Hospital, as opposed to Mengo Hospital, in 1921. By 1927, the Uganda branch of the BMA had started to hold regular scientific meetings, and mission doctors maintained an active presence until the 1940s at least.[71] A report on the inter-territorial meeting of the East African Branches of the BMA, held in Kampala in May 1936, described how mission and government doctors came together to discuss topics as diverse as the mental adjustment of Africans, urban and rural plague, and the frequency of trachoma in natives.[72] While these discussions could lead to extended debates between individual mission and government doctors, these activities nevertheless underscored an implicit *esprit de corps* as medical colleagues and 'experts'.

The doctors at Mengo Hospital remained influential in official government circles until the 1930s, but requests for advice on sanitation, hygiene, and town planning appear to have come more out of respect for Albert Cook than out of any feeling that Mengo Hospital still retained exceptional insight into local health and disease conditions. Indeed, as Cook withdrew from medical practice at Mengo Hospital in 1934, so did the regular requests for advice and assistance. By the mid-1930s, the influence that Mengo Hospital had previously enjoyed was on the wane, and changes in government legislation on patient fees and charges prompted the first of several financial crises.[73] In 1934, Robert Stones, the new head doctor of Mengo Hospital, finalised an arrangement for a government grant to support medical work at the hospital. While the mission doctors were to remain free to continue ward services, the grant came with other conditions, including a note to the effect that Schofield would ideally not play any leading role in the hospital. Having co-opted him as a half-time DMO in Toro during the 1920s and found him 'difficult', the government was anxious not to deal with him again.[74]

Finally, in 1939, the Colonial Medical Service set out its views on the future of Mengo Hospital. With the addition of 300 new beds at Mulago Hospital planned for 1940, it was anticipated that 'the need for Mengo Hospital as a general hospital would then pass away'.[75] Mengo Hospital, as Jack Cook and Stones reported back to the CMS, might then serve one of three purposes:

a. That the Hospital should function as a hostel for the enlarged Mulago and the University that is to be.
b. That it should be a training school, recognised by Government, for the training of nurses during their first years.
c. That it should undertake certain specialized activities which Government never intends to take up, such as Orthopaedic work, Tuberculosis work, Leprosy etc.[76]

The emphasis of the Colonial Medical Service on curative as well as preventive medicine had shifted the relationship between mission and government doctors to the point where missionary input was no longer required. With it, the high level of collaboration that had characterised Western medical practice in early colonial Uganda ceased almost entirely.

Conclusion

Michael Jennings has argued that historians of medical missions have tended 'to define "missionary medicine" as something peculiar to the Christian mission', stressing its evangelical and Christian theological underpinnings rather than the ways mission doctors responded to wider trends in medicine.[77] These mission doctors, as Jennings has pointed out, 'had the same training that all doctors underwent, read articles in medical journals, were kept informed of latest developments, and participated in research trials of new drugs'.[78] CMS doctors in Uganda, too, were not isolated from wider intellectual communities, and played an active role in education and research both in Uganda and further afield. These activities brought together mission and government doctors as professional colleagues and experts, and in turn shaped what both 'missionary medicine' and 'colonial medicine' could offer to their patients.

The complexity of the relationship between mission and government doctors in early colonial Uganda means that neither missionary nor colonial medicine should be considered in isolation. In this period, mission doctors and colonial medical officers were granted a considerable degree of autonomy in their everyday medical practice. As a result, the sharing of specialist knowledge, language skills, technical equipment, and personnel was surprisingly non-contentious. What was deemed to be appropriate 'missionary' as opposed to 'government' medical work was rarely, if ever, well defined, as mission and government doctors alike consulted and collaborated on individual patients and matters of policy. Indeed, missionary and colonial medicine were defined as much in relation to each other as they were within the broader context of general medical provision in Uganda.

Any history of missionary medicine inevitably touches on questions of power. Missionaries have frequently been accused of promoting 'cultural imperialism'; acting as vanguards for colonial overrule and as agents for imperial expansion.[79] Certainly, for much of the colonial period, the Colonial Medical Service in Uganda relied on missionaries to share their knowledge of local health and disease conditions and to implement medical services in areas it was unable or unwilling to administer. Yet, while mission doctors wielded a considerable amount of power, they were hardly unproblematic 'agents of Empire', nor were they ignorant of the implications of their collaboration. These missionaries, as Jeffrey Cox has argued for the Indian context, 'struggled with the conflict between universalist Christian religious values and the imperial context of those values'.[80] Missionaries who engaged in government service in Uganda expressed tension, anxiety, and confusion over discrepancies between the rules set out by the CMS and the practical realities of practising medicine in colonial Africa. Money, facilities, and intellectual communities were as important to the medical work of mission doctors as was their belief in God.

In many ways this chapter has presented a one-sided history. By focusing on the relationship between missionary and government doctors in their everyday practice, it has missed out one group of historical actors: patients and their families. These are an essential part of any history of Western medicine, not least because, for most, mission and government hospitals were peripheral agents of health-care. Families continued to care for their sick in their own ways, and to make decisions about treatment that were unrelated to either government or mission policy. This was due in part to the limited reach of Western medicine – Singo County, for example, had by 1935 only one government-run dispensary to serve an estimated population of 70,000, spread over 2,734 square miles.[81] But it was also because those families who did engage with Western medicine did so largely on their own terms, and with their own expectations and priorities in mind. As John Orley, anthropologist and psychiatrist, noted on patient choices in Uganda, 'Africans, being pragmatists, looked for a system that worked, and if one traditional remedy failed then another could be tried and so on until eventually Western medical treatment could also be given its chance'.[82]

This vast, and as yet inadequately explored, area of history is well beyond the scope of this chapter.[83] However, a few examples from the patient case notes of Mengo Hospital are instructive. Nakoli M. was admitted to Mengo Hospital in 1929, having been found walking around Kampala by the police. Although he had been originally sent to Mulago Hospital, the doctors there had been unwilling to deal with him, and had passed him over to Mengo Hospital, where Alma Downes-Shaw, along with medical student Y.K. Tabamwenda, diagnosed Nakoli with acute mania. They prescribed multiple doses of potassium bromide on a daily basis, a drug used widely in asylums in the United Kingdom and India to sedate patients. After a month there was still no improvement in his condition and he was '[t]aken away against wish of the Doctor'. Nakoli maintained that he had been 'given poison mixed in water by a native', and it was perhaps a remedy for this poison that his relatives wished to find elsewhere.[84] More detail is evident in the case notes for Erina W., who was admitted to Mengo Hospital by R.Y. Stones in 1935, following a history of violence, hysteria, insomnia, and 'talking nonsense'. Towards the end of her twenty-day stay at the hospital, Erina took a dislike to her husband and the head hospital girl. Shortly after, and perhaps suspecting that the hospital staff were turning Erina against him, her husband removed her from the hospital.[85] In these cases, as in many others, families remained unconvinced about the ability of either mission or government doctors to relieve the suffering of their relatives. Indeed, it was partly the belief that Western medicine would be successful only when it was practised by African medical practitioners that fuelled attempts to train African medical practitioners, which both mission and government doctors sought to control.[86]

In Uganda in the early twentieth-first century the words 'history of medicine' remain synonymous with Albert Cook and Mengo Hospital. All medical students passing through Makerere University study in the Albert Cook Memorial Library at Mulago Hospital, which still houses Mengo Hospital's earliest patient case notes. The history that is woven into the educational lives of each generation of doctors sees missionaries as pioneers in Western medicine, setting up the foundations from which the government eventually took over. Yet it also perhaps acts as a statement of independence – as a reminder of the extent to which African medical practitioners have moved away from the colonial past, and have transformed their own profession.

Acknowledgements

This research was funded by a Wellcome Trust doctoral studentship, with support from the British Institute in Eastern Africa and Jesus College, Oxford. My thanks go to Anna Greenwood, Ryan Johnson, and the anonymous reviewer for their helpful comments.

Notes

1 This point has also been made in Jan Kuhanen, *Poverty, Health and Reproduction in Early Colonial Uganda*, Joensuu, Finland, University of Joensuu Publications in the Humanities 37, 2005, p. 247

2 This literature includes: Ann Beck, *A History of the British Medical Administration of East Africa: 1900–1950*, Cambridge, MA, Harvard University Press, 1970; W.D. Foster, 'Doctor Albert Cook and the Early Days of the Church Missionary Society's Medical Mission to Uganda', *Medical History*, 12, 4, 1968, pp. 325–43; W.D. Foster, *The Early History of Scientific Medicine in Uganda*, Nairobi, East African Literature Bureau, 1970; Kirk Arden Hoppe, *Lords of the Fly: Sleeping Sickness Control in British East Africa, 1900–1960*, Westport, CT, Praeger, 2003; Kuhanen, *Poverty, Health and Reproduction*; Carol Summers, 'Intimate Colonialism: The Imperial Production of Reproduction in Uganda, 1907–1925', *Signs*, 16, 4, 1991, pp. 787–807; Michael William Tuck, 'Syphilis, Sexuality, and Social Control: A History of Venereal Disease in Colonial Uganda', unpublished PhD thesis, Northwestern University, 1997; Megan Vaughan, *Curing Their Ills: Colonial Power and African Illness*, Cambridge, Polity Press, 1991; Kathleen Vongsathorn, '"First and Foremost the Evangelist"? Mission and Government Priorities for the Treatment of Leprosy in Uganda, 1927–48', *Journal of Eastern African Studies*, 6, 3, 2012, pp. 544–60; Diane L. Zeller, 'The Establishment of Western Medicine in Buganda', unpublished PhD thesis, Columbia University, 1971

3 Summers, 'Intimate Colonialism', p. 803

4 John Iliffe, *East African Doctors: A History of the Modern Profession*, Kampala, Fountain Publishers, 2002
5 Anna Crozier, *Practising Colonial Medicine: The Colonial Medical Service in British East Africa*, New York, I.B. Tauris & Co. Ltd, 2007, pp. 60–1
6 Vongsathorn, '"First and Foremost the Evangelist"?'
7 For an excellent review of the ways in which the historiography of medical missions has been plagued by generalisations and misconceptions, see especially Michael Jennings, '"A Matter of Vital Importance": The Place of the Medical Mission in Maternal and Child Healthcare in Tanganyika, 1919–39', in David Hardiman (ed.), *Healing Bodies, Saving Souls: Medical Missions in Asia and Africa*, Amsterdam and New York, Rodopi, 2006; Michael Jennings, '"This Mysterious and Intangible Enemy": Health and Disease Amongst the Early UMCA Missionaries, 1860–1918', *Social History of Medicine*, 15, 1, 2002, pp. 65–87
8 These have included W.R. Billington, 'Albert Cook: A Biographical Note', *East African Medical Journal*, 10, 28, 1951, pp. 397–422; Foster, *The Early History of Scientific Medicine*; H.C. Trowell, 'The Medical Pioneers and Explorers of East Africa', *East African Medical Journal*, 34, 8, 1957, pp. 417–30
9 There is certainly room for a history of Catholic medical missions in Uganda, and in particular the history of Rubaga Hospital. Summers, 'Intimate Colonialism', p. 799; Vongsathorn, '"First and Foremost the Evangelist"?'.
10 On the early history of Mengo Hospital, see especially W.D. Foster, *The Church Missionary Society and Modern Medicine in Uganda the Life of Sir Albert Cook, K.C.M.G., 1870–1951*, Newhaven, CT, Newhaven Press, 1978; Foster, 'Doctor Albert Cook'
11 Rhodes House Library, Oxford (RHL) Micr.Afr.609(4) Papers of J.N.P. Davies, Medical Report for the Year Ending March 31, 1903
12 RHL Micr.Afr.609(4) Papers of J.N.P. Davies, Medical Report for the Year Ending March 31, 1903
13 Albert Ruskin Cook, *Uganda Memories, 1897–1940*, Kampala, Uganda Society, 1945, p. 1; J.H. Cook, 'Notes on Cases of "Sleeping Sickness" Occurring in the Uganda Protectorate', *Journal of Tropical Medicine*, 1901, p. 237; Douglas M. Haynes, 'Framing Tropical Disease in London: Patrick Manson, *Filaria Perstans*, and the Uganda Sleeping Sickness Epidemic, 1891–1902', *Social History of Medicine*, 13, 3, 2000, pp. 467–93, pp. 485–7
14 See, for example, Albert Cook Memorial Library, Makerere University, Uganda (ACMM) Sir Albert Cook Records, Mengo Hospital Correspondence, 1897–1963 (MHC) letter from C.A. Wiggins to Dr Cook, 23 December 1914; ACMH MHC letter from J.M. Collyns to Dr Cook, 22 July 1915; ACMH MHC letter from G.O. Stratham to Dr Cook, 14 February 1916
15 ACMH MHC letter from C.J. Baker, Medical Sanitary Officer, to Albert Cook, 31 August 1916
16 ACMH MHC letter from L. Allworth to A. Cook, 2 March 1914
17 University of Birmingham Special Collections (UoBSC) G3 A7/O 1919 Uganda Mission Outgoing Correspondence 1919, fo.35, letter from Albert Cook to Dr Lankester, 18 February 1919
18 See, for example, ACMM MHC, letter from R. van Someren to Dr Cook, 8 May 1915. Such was the popularity of Albert Cook in particular, that on his retirement in 1934 mission authorities feared that his withdrawal into private practice would necessitate the closure of Mengo Hospital altogether. UoBSC G3 A7/O 1934, Uganda Mission Outgoing Correspondence 1934, fo.40, letter from Bishop of Uganda to Rev. H.D. Hooper, London, 13 March 1934
19 UoBSC Acc. 514, Papers of Winifred Annie Milnes-Walker, Report of the CMS Mengo Hospital, Uganda, 1897–1937; E.N. Cook, 'The Adventures of an X-Ray', *Mercy and Truth*, 276, 1920, pp. 277–81
20 J.H. Cook, 'A Year's Hospital Work in Central Africa', *Church Missionary Review*, 66, 796, 1915, pp. 482–6, p. 485
21 On the Uganda branch of the BMA, see Crozier, *Practising Colonial Medicine*,

pp. 96–7; J.N.P. Davies, 'The History of the Uganda Branch of the British Medical Association, 1913 to 1932', *East African Medical Journal*, 31, 3, 1954, pp. 93–9

22   Davies, 'The History of the Uganda Branch', p. 94

23   See, for example, ACMM MHC, letter from R. van Someren to Dr Cook, 22 July 1915

24   J.H. Cook, 'Missionaries and War Service', *Mercy and Truth*, 226, 1915, pp. 326–8, p. 328

25   T. Beidelman, *Colonial Evangelism: A Socio-Historical Study of an East African Mission at the Grassroots*, Bloomington, IN, Indiana University Press, 1982, p. 76; David Hardiman, 'Introduction', in David Hardiman (ed.), *Healing Bodies, Saving Souls: Medical Missions in Asia and Africa*, Amsterdam and New York, Rodopi, 2006, p. 25

26   Hardiman, 'Introduction', pp. 18–20

27   On the expansion of government medical services, see especially: The National Archives, UK (TNA) CO 536/140 History of Ugda Medical Reforms; TNA CO 536/129 Medical Department. Coordination of Services and General Reorganisation; Beck, *A History of the British Medical Administration*; Crozier, *Practising Colonial Medicine*

28   The districts and years served were: L.E.S. Sharp (Kigezi, 1921–29); E.N. Cook (Toro, 1923–24); A.T. Schofield (Toro, 1924–25); A.C. Stanley Smith (Kigezi, temporarily, 1925)

29   J.H. Cook, *9th Annual Report of Toro Medical Mission*, Torquay, C. Bendle, St. Mary Church Printing Works, 1911. The Roman Catholics maintained a small medical mission at Virunga, but Ashton Bond was the only doctor in the area

30   J.H. Cook, *9th Annual Report*, 1911

31   Uganda Protectorate, *Annual Medical and Sanitary Report for the Year Ended 31st December, 1919*, Entebbe, Government Printer, Uganda, 1920, p. 13

32   UoBSC G3 A7/O 1920 111–end Uganda Mission Outgoing Correspondence 1920, fo.197, letter from Ashton Bond to George Manley, 12 October 1920

33   UoBSC G3 A7/O 1920 1–110 Uganda Mission Outgoing Correspondence 1920, fo.69, letter from F. Rowling to George Manley, 17 February 1920; UoBSC G3 A7/O 1920 111–end, fo.197, letter from Ashton Bond to George Manley, 12 October 1920

34   UoBSC G3 A7/O 1921 Uganda Mission Outgoing Correspondence 1921, fo.68, letter from Ashton Bond to George Manley, 3 May 1921

35   UoBSC G3 A7/O 1920 111–end Uganda Mission Outgoing Correspondence 1920, fo.198, letter from Rowling to Manley, 19 October 1920; UoBSC G3 A7/O 1920 111–end Uganda Mission Outgoing Correspondence 1920, fo.199, letter from Rowling to Manley, 21 October 1920

36   UoBSC G3 A7/O 1920 111–end Uganda Mission Outgoing Correspondence 1920, fo.197, letter from Ashton Bond to George Manley, 12 October 1920

37   UoBSC G3 A7/O 1920 111–end Uganda Mission Outgoing Correspondence 1920, 1922 saw a 5% reduction in missionary stipends in Uganda, on which medical and non-medical missionaries at Namirembe noted that any more would result in serious hardship. UoBSC G3 A7/O 1922 Uganda Mission Outgoing Correspondence 1922, fo.80, letter from H. Boulton Ladbury to Mr Manley, 17 July 1922

38   UoBSC G3 A7/O 1920 111–end, fo.198, letter from Rowling to Manley, 19 October 1920

39   UoBSC G3 A7/O 1920 1–110, fo.28, 'Minute of Medical Committee, January 27, 1920'

40   UoBSC G3 A7/L4 1919–1926 Uganda Mission Letterbook 1919–26, pp. 106–7, letter from George Manley to Mr Ladbury, 9 June 1921; UoBSC G3 A7/O 1921, fo.63, letter from C.A. Wiggins to Dr Sharp, 21 March 1921; UoBSC G3 A7/O 1921, fo.83, letter from A.C. Stanley Smith to 'My dear Ruanda friend', 7 May 1921

41   UoBSC G3 A7/O 1921, fo.68, letter from Ashton Bond to George Manley, 3 May 1921

42   UoBSC G3 A7/O 1921, fo.68, letter from Ashton Bond to George Manley, 3 May 1921

43   See Crozier, *Practising Colonial Medicine*, p. 91; Ryan Johnson, '"An All-white

Institution": Defending Private Practice and the Formation of the West African Medical Staff', *Medical History*, 54, 2010, pp. 237–54

44 Kabale District Archives (KDA) Medical General 1921–5, letter from Ag. PMO to Sharp, 22 September 1922

45 KDA Medical General 1921–5, memo from PMO to PC Western Province, 20 October 1921

46 KDA Medical General 1921–5, letter from Sharp to DC Kabale, 28 April 1921

47 UoBSC G3 A7/O 1919, fo.166, letter from Sharp to Manley, 24 December 1919

48 KDA Medical General 1921–5, letter from P.W. Cooper to PMO, 22 September 1922

49 E.N. Cook was in 1923, and Schofield in 1925. Mountains of the Moon University Archives, Uganda (MMU) MED 1079(295) Medical Policy

50 UoBSC G3 A7/O 1934, fo.106, letter from A.T. Schofield to Rev. Hooper, 3 October 1934

51 UoBSC G3 A7/O 1923, Uganda Mission Outgoing Correspondence 1923, fo.108, Medical Sub-Conference Minutes, 6 November 1923; UoBSC G3 A7/O 1934, fo.106, letter from A.T. Schofield to Rev. Hooper, 3 October 1934

52 KDA Medical General 1921–8, Kabale, 22 March 1923

53 KDA Medical General 1921–5, letter from PC Western Province to PMO, 24 March 1925

54 KDA Medical General 1921–5, letter from PC Western Province to PMO, 24 March 1925

55 KDA Medical General 1921–5, letter from PC Western Province to PMO, 24 March 1925

56 KDA Medical General 1921–5, letter from PMO to PC Western Province, 14 April 1925

57 Uganda Protectorate, *Annual Medical and Sanitary Report for the Year Ended 31st December, 1925*, Entebbe, Government Printer, Uganda, 1926, p. 21

58 KDA Medical General, letter from Chief Secretary to Sharp, 7 January 1929; KDA Medical General 1921–5, letter from PC Western Province to PMO, 24 March 1925; KDA Medical General 1921–5, letter from PMO to PC Western Province, 14 April 1925

59 UoBSC G3 A7/O 1923, fo.109, Medical Sub-Conference Minutes, 6 November 1923

60 On medical work in Uganda, see especially Iliffe, *East African Doctors*; Audrey W. Williams, 'The History of Mulago Hospital and the Makerere College Medical School', *East African Medical Journal*, 29, 7, 1952, pp. 253–63

61 E.N. Cook, 'A Medical Mission in War Time', *Mercy and Truth*, 216, 1914, pp. 392–4, p. 394

62 See Iliffe, *East African Doctors*, ch. 3; Maryinez Lyons, 'The Power to Heal: African Medical Auxiliaries in Colonial Belgian Congo and Uganda', in Dagmar Engels and Shula Marks (eds.), *Contesting Colonial Hegemony: State and Society in Africa and India*, London, British Academic Press, 1994. On African medical practitioners elsewhere, see especially Anne Digby, 'Early Black Doctors in South Africa', *Journal of African History*, 46, 2005, pp. 427–54; Walima T. Kalusa, 'Language, Medical Auxiliaries, and the Re-interpretation of Missionary Medicine in Colonial Mwinilunga, Zambia, 1922–51', *Journal of Eastern African Studies*, 1, 1, 2007, pp. 57–78; Johnson, '"An All-white Institution"'

63 ACMM MHC, copy of letter from Albert Cook to Ernest Cook, 13 April 1928

64 ACMM MHC, copy of letter from Albert Cook to Ernest Cook, 13 April 1928

65 ACMM MHC, letter from Ernest Cook to Albert Cook, 22 April 1928

66 Crozier, *Practising Colonial Medicine*, p. 60

67 Hardiman has made this point more generally on missionary medicine in Hardiman, 'Introduction', p. 20

68 UoBSC G3 A7/O 1928 Uganda Mission Outgoing Correspondence 1928, fo.22, letter from Boulton Ladbury to Hooper, 20 February 1928

69 ACMM MHC, letter from Claude Marshall, Senior Medical Officer, Buganda, to Dr Cook, 10 October 1925; ACMM MHC, letter from Scott to Stones, 5 June 1935; UoBSC Acc. 514, F5 Newspaper Cuttings, 1947–66, 'Dr. R.Y. Stones … The Man

from London who Became the Africans' Friend: The Humble Christian', *Uganda Argus*, nd.; UoBSC Acc. 514, F5 Newspaper Cuttings, 1947–66, Report of the CMS Mengo Hospital, Uganda, 1897–1937

70 Tuck, 'Syphilis, Sexuality, and Social Control', p. 229

71 Davies, 'The History of the Uganda Branch', p. 97

72 'Meetings of Branches and Divisions', *Supplement to the British Medical Journal*, 11 July 1936, p. 29

73 In 1938, for example, a change in the medical regulations meant that only registered physicians could distribute poisonous medicines, including arsenic and mercury, the main anti-syphilis medications. This removed a large proportion of medical mission income. Tuck, 'Syphilis, Sexuality, and Social Control', p. 224

74 ACMM MHC, letter from Scott to Stones, December 1934

75 ACMM MHC, letter from the Bishop's House, Kampala, to the Chief Secretary, 18 April 1939

76 ACMM MHC, letter from the Bishop's House, Kampala, to the Chief Secretary, 18 April 1939

77 Jennings, '"A Matter of Vital Importance"', pp. 229–30. Ryan Johnson has reinforced this point in Ryan Johnson, 'Colonial Mission and Imperial Tropical Medicine: Livingstone College, London, 1893–1914', *Social History of Medicine*, 23, 3, 2010, pp. 549–66

78 Jennings, '"A Matter of Vital Importance"', pp. 229–30

79 Jeffrey Cox, 'Audience and Exclusion at the Margins of Imperial History', *Women's History Review*, 3, 4, 1994, pp. 501–14; Andrew Porter, '"Cultural Imperialism" and protestant Missionary Enterprise, 1780–1914', *Journal of Imperial and Commonwealth History*, 25, 3, 1997, pp. 367–91; Brian Stanley, *The Bible and the Flag: Protestant Missions and British Imperialism in the Nineteenth and Twentieth Centuries*, Leicester, Apollos, 1990

80 Jeffrey Cox, *Imperial Fault Lines: Christianity and Colonial Power in India, 1818–1940*, Stanford, CA, Stanford University Press, 2002, p. 6

81 Zeller, 'The Establishment of Western Medicine', p. 276

82 John Orley, 'Indigenous Concepts of Disease and Their Interaction with Scientific Medicine', in E.E. Sabben-Clare, D.J. Bradley, and K. Kirkwood (eds.), *Health in Tropical Africa during the Colonial Period: Based on the Proceedings of a Symposium Held at New College, Oxford, 21–23 March 1977*, Oxford, Clarendon Press, 1980, p. 127

83 A good starting point for such a study in Uganda would be Zeller, 'The Establishment of Western Medicine'.

84 ACMM Mengo Hospital Case Notes (MHCN), 1929, Volume 5, Case No. 1375

85 ACMM MHCN, 1935, Volume 2, Case No. 620

86 I have written about this in relation to psychiatric training. See Yolana Pringle, 'Investigating "Mass Hysteria" in Early Postcolonial Uganda: Benjamin H. Kagwa, East African Psychiatry, and the Gisu', *Journal of the History of Medicine and Allied Sciences*, 70, 1, 2015, pp. 105–36

CHAPTER THREE

The government medical service and British missions in colonial Malawi, c. 1891–1940: crucial collaboration, hidden conflicts

Markku Hokkanen

As Megan Vaughan has pointed out, for most of the colonial period in Africa, Christian missions 'provided vastly more medical care than did colonial states'.[1] Indeed, from the outset of European colonial rule, most imperial states left the provision of the majority of education and healthcare to Christian missions.[2]

In colonial Malawi, missionary medicine preceded British rule by nearly two decades, making it a crucial site for investigating relations and interactions between missions and the state.[3] As Vaughan and others have shown, there were notable differences as well as common ground between missionary and secular discourses of African illnesses and Western medicine in colonial Africa.[4] The focus of this chapter is on the connections and exchanges that took place within the realms of medicine and public health between the colonial administration (particularly its medical department) and the British missions of Livingstonia, Blantyre and the Universities' Mission to Central Africa (UMCA).[5]

In his assessment of the early colonial medical service in Malawi, Colin Baker presents a generally sympathetic account of an under-resourced medical department that gradually expanded its services to the African population and provided a form of public medical service to colonial subjects (before the National Health Service had been established in Britain).[6] By contrast, Charles Good's more recent appraisal of colonial medicine in Malawi is highly critical. Notably, in discussing the reasons for this, Good highlights the colonial government's limited cooperation and support for missionary medicine, arguing that formal collaboration between the two groups was largely limited to the treatment of leprosy patients.[7]

In order to better understand the contexts in which Western

medicine was practised in British Africa, both formal and informal modes of cooperation (and conflict) must be examined.[8] This chapter discusses the ties that connected missionary physicians and the Colonial Medical Service: public health campaigns, the division of labour, the exchanges of knowledge and materials and issues raised surrounding the ownership of African medical education. Western medical practice in Malawi has largely been viewed as dominated by missionary physicians until the First World War, after which government medical services became increasingly prominent. While this overview is generally accurate, it over-simplifies the reality that witnessed a long history of many connections, relations and exchanges between government and mission medicine. This chapter seeks to explore these relations and interactions in order to illustrate the formal and informal forms of cooperation, contestation and conflict. Despite many differences, colonial and missionary medicine were intertwined, with each benefitting from the other's cooperative co-existence.

Missions and colonial administration

The first permanent mission in Malawi was the Free Church of Scotland's Livingstonia Mission. Livingstonia's first medical missionary, Robert Laws, arrived with the pioneer party in 1875. Laws, a qualified doctor, headed the mission for many years and became a respected missionary statesman: his voluminous correspondence remains a valuable source for investigations into mission–government relations.[9] The second permanent missionary establishment in Malawi was the Blantyre Mission of the Church of Scotland, founded in 1876 in the Shire Highlands. Significantly, both Scottish missions referred to their doctors as Medical Officers, a practice which was to be adopted by most government medical services in Africa, emphasising their official authority. The English Anglican Universities' Mission to Central Africa (UMCA) returned to Malawi in 1882 (after its first failed attempt in the 1860s), and established a station on Likoma Island near the eastern shore of the Lake Malawi.[10] In 1900, both the UMCA and Livingstonia operated across areas that were both on and beyond the borders of the fledgling British Central Africa Protectorate. Both held a practical monopoly over the practice of Western medicine in their respective borders.[11] By contrast, the Blantyre mission concentrated its work at the heart of the new protectorate in the southern region of Malawi.

The Scottish missions and churches played a crucial part in lobbying for the establishment of a British Protectorate over the Lake Nyasa region.[12] After the establishment of the Protectorate, the Blantyre

Mission in particular clashed with Harry Johnston's administration. Missionaries criticised Johnston's military campaigns against African rulers, his often brutal methods of tax collection and the treatment of Africans more generally under his tenure. The missionaries at Blantyre also pointed out that the general population received little in return for their tax and labour contributions. They pressed the government to give greater medical attention to Africans.[13]

Johnston had set out to establish the British Protectorate in Central Africa with meagre resources, initially funded by Cecil Rhodes's British South Africa Company. In the early 1890s the British Central Africa Protectorate was established through a series of treaties and 'small wars'.[14] Johnston's administration employed only a handful of doctors. In 1891, the entire medical services budget was £250 – less than the salary of a single Scottish missionary doctor. The first permanent government Medical Officer (MO), Wordsworth Poole, set up his practice in Zomba, the new capital, in 1895. Mortality rates for MOs were high in the 1890s: by 1901 four government doctors had died. Nevertheless, medical personnel were still recruited to the region and by 1910 the annual budget allocated to the medical department had increased to £9,000. On the back of these funds, the government established its main hospital in Zomba.[15] Despite relatively meagre resources, the medical department was the second largest of the colonial administration, with government medical practitioners largely operating in the Shire Highlands and lower Shire river region.[16] By the First World War, the Colonial Medical Service had considerably expanded its services in the southern part of the country, which represented the hub of the colonial economy.

The government first began to support missionary medicine in Blantyre, where a major mission hospital, St Luke's Hospital, was established in the late 1890s. In the early 1900s, the government funded two of the hospital's beds (at the cost of £20 per annum). In 1906 the government additionally gave £50 to support five beds in a smaller mission hospital in Zomba, and two years later this hospital was put under government control, most likely because it was deemed more fitting to have a government-run hospital in the capital.[17] Nevertheless the Blantyre Mission continued to dominate medical services for Africans in the commercial centre of the Protectorate. In 1939, the government paid an annual subsidy of £600 to the Blantyre hospital. During the interwar period, the Church of Scotland mission also received payment for the upkeep of its Asiatic Hospital in Blantyre.[18]

As in other African colonial territories, before the First World War, the tiny Colonial Medical Service in Malawi focused its efforts on the health of government employees and on high-profile campaigns against major epidemic diseases. During this period, missions clearly remained the primary source of Western medicine for the majority of the African population.[19]

In terms of in-patient numbers, St Luke's hospital in Blantyre was by far the largest hospital in Malawi for most of the early colonial period: as early as 1897 over 300 patients were admitted. This popularity grew, with hospital records for 1903 indicating that over 800 in-patients were treated during that year.[20] Similarly, between 1904 and 1911, the UMCA hospital in Likoma was the second largest hospital in Malawi. In the north, the central hospital in Livingstonia became a major regional healthcare facility during the 1910s and 1920s.[21]

Perhaps unsurprisingly, in the Shire Highlands, missionary medicine tended to focus on African male workers. A clear majority of the early in-patients at Blantyre were male. As Rennick has argued, the colonial settlers became important 'refereeing agents' for the Blantyre hospital, and mission medicine took on an active role in the control and examination of African labour. Many of those treated were migrant labourers. The administration also became a referring agent for mission hospitals: in Blantyre in the early 1900s and in Zomba between 1903 and 1908.[22]

African patients were frequently referred to mission hospitals by government agents. There were fewer recommendations from missions to send patients to colonial hospitals, with the notable exception of those who were deemed to be 'lunatics'. The history of the movement of the insane is indicative of broader moral concerns over offering faith-based care to members of society deemed socially problematic. Since the early 1900s missions had strongly pressed the government to establish an asylum in the territory, a request that was realised only in 1910 with the establishment of the poorly resourced Zomba Asylum (1910), which was initially part of the Central Prison. Even after the establishment of this asylum, however, it was evident that missionaries wanted 'incurable' cases to be taken care of by the state, thus removing problematic elements of society from mission communities. In 1913, Laws told the Legislative Council that he spoke for all medical missionaries when he expressed relief that there was now a place to which dangerous cases could be sent. Furthermore, the mission connection with the Zomba Asylum undoubtedly contributed to the way in which secular colonial medicine assessed African insanity. In 1935, Nyasaland MOs Shelly and Watson concluded in their study of Zomba inmates that increasing contact with civilisation, education and Christianity was dangerous for African mental health, thereby inferring (among other things) that is was better that the African insane were removed from missionary influences.[23]

Government medical services expanded considerably during the interwar years. In 1921, the government medical staff treated 19,000 African cases; and by 1937, 729,000 cases were treated, with medical expenditure increasing to £53,000 in 1938.[24] Despite this expansion, the Director of Medical and Sanitary Services reported in 1939 that 'the Medical Department has not yet been able to make contact with the African population in the full measure necessary to gain its confidence'. In the 1930s, government services were still very much focused on the southern part of the Protectorate.[25] In many rural areas, mission hospitals and dispensaries remained the only scattered outposts of Western medicine.

Indeed, so scarce were government medical facilities in rural areas that missionary doctors were informally relied upon to treat government officials and their families when they were posted to, or travelling in, remote areas. This trend was regarded as significant enough to warrant an appeal in 1923 from the Nyasaland government to the Colonial Office to put in place more formal procedures to allow the Governor to pay non-official doctors for the treatment of officers at remote outstations.[26] Illustratively, in 1925, the Indian Sub-Assistant Surgeon in charge of the government hospital at Mzimba, Northern Province, suffered a stroke and was taken to the nearest doctor, Agnes Fraser (Livingstonia) at Loudon.[27]

Occasionally, doctors and nurses moved from mission to government service.[28] For ambitious mission doctors, colonial medical posts could offer research opportunities and contractual perks, but movements of personnel were also motivated by personal frustration or by conflicts within the missions.[29] In 1897, for example, David Kerr Cross of Livingstonia switched to a government post, a move that took place against a backdrop of enduring tensions and conflicts within his mission. Sir Harry Johnston clearly appreciated Cross's change of allegiance, and quoted him as a medical expert in his book, *British Central Africa*.[30]

Similarly, in 1903, Samuel Norris of the Blantyre Mission joined the Colonial Medical Service. Norris was at least partly motivated by a desire to spend more time researching tropical medicine, having been clearly dissatisfied with the opportunities presented by his position in Blantyre. According to Rennick, Norris 'never fully internalised and fulfilled the evangelical aspects of the medical missionaries' role'.[31]

Despite these cases, however, there was relatively little mobility of doctors between mission and government service. Mission and government doctors in Malawi were largely distinct groups, which were nevertheless connected through the British medical profession, education and the small elite circles within which Europeans in the Protectorate operated. From 1926 onwards, mission and government doctors met regularly at meetings of the Nyasaland Medical Council. Officially at least, cooperation was regarded as a success, with the Director of Medical Services (DMS) admitting in 1940 that, through advice and cooperation, the missionaries had 'helped to shape the medical policy of the country'.[32]

As Baker points out, the 1906 Registration of Medical Practitioners Ordinance of Nyasaland was 'highly biased' towards British qualifications.[33] An early exception to the rule was Daniel Malekebu of the Providence Industrial Mission (PIM), a Malawian who had obtained his medical qualifications in the United States. Malekebu was viewed with some suspicion by the authorities, probably because his mission had been at the heart of the Chilembwe Rising in 1915. In 1927, Malekebu's status as a mission doctor was considered by the highest levels of the colonial government, with the Executive Council ultimately agreeing that he was eligible for registration under the Ordinance.[34] Simply put, the colonial medical department tacitly recognised the medical work of the three major British missions. By 1940, the Dutch Reformed Church and Seventh Day Adventists were also acknowledged for their medical facilities, although the Catholic missions and Malekebu's PIM were not.[35]

The important question of the extent to which Malawians themselves differentiated between colonial and missionary medicine is beyond the scope of this chapter.[36] However, it seems that in the early colonial period, and in village communities with little direct contact with hospitals or dispensaries, Western medicine was generally categorised as a medicine of the whites (*mankhwala achizungu* in chiChewa). Among those with direct experience of Western medicine, people quickly formed opinions about medical personnel and hospitals: by the interwar period, Malawians spoke dismissively of 'boys' medicine' (*mtela achiboyi*) and condemned hospitals with low standards.[37] In the end, whether delivered by representatives of the Church or the state, assessments of Western medicine crucially depended on African patients' experiences of the healing skills of the medical personnel, expressions of goodwill and the cost of treatment.

Cooperation in epidemics: smallpox, sleeping sickness, bubonic plague

Epidemic diseases required a coordinated response from missions and the administration. In the Shire Highlands, Blantyre Mission and the government were united in their goal of protecting the region from epidemics that were a threat to Africans and Europeans alike. The oldest of the major epidemic diseases was smallpox, which had been known and feared in South-Central Africa in the pre-colonial era. In the Shire valley at least, variolation was practised in the nineteenth century before the arrival of Europeans, demonstrating that the principle of vaccination was not alien to local societies.[38] In any case, it is certain that missionaries introduced Western vaccination to Malawi before the establishment of colonial rule, with evidence showing that Laws had access to a supply of lymph as early as 1875, and that by 1883 vaccinations had been carried out in both Livingstonia and Blantyre.[39]

Smallpox vaccination was one of the most efficient tools in demonstrating efficacy that early missionary and colonial doctors possessed. Correspondingly, it was much sought after. In Northern Ngoniland, for example, it was one form of Western medicine for which people were eagerly willing to pay, even though the process of vaccinations was often hindered by the failure of the lymph supply.[40] Furthermore, large-scale campaigns required vaccinators, and at the turn of the century missions could provide the crucial African and European personnel that the government lacked.

In the Shire Highlands, the initiative for collaborative vaccination campaigns came from the Blantyre Mission, where Neil Macvicar had established a dynamic central hospital and a ground-breaking training programme for African medical assistants. The government MOs joined the campaign in 1899. Blantyre had trained African vaccinators and medical assistants, such as Harry Kambwiri, who for their part enabled the vaccination of tens of thousands of people in the Shire Highlands. By 1903, smallpox prevention measures in Southern Malawi were deemed largely successful. The colonial administration gave full credit to medical missionaries for this evident success, and especially to the Blantyre Mission (which had reportedly vaccinated 60,000 people in the Blantyre district between 1900 and 1902).[41] For its part, the UMCA was also important within the history of vaccination provision in Malawi, especially in the border zone between the British Protectorate and German East Africa (1899–1900).[42]

After smallpox epidemics reoccurred in 1908, the administration issued a Vaccination Ordinance, which imposed compulsory vaccination and prohibited variolation. It appeared that implementation of this ordinance relied upon the successful cooperation between faith-based and secular medical groups. In the Legislative Council, Alexander Hetherwick of Blantyre heartily advocated compulsory vaccination, praised mission–government cooperation and voiced suspicions that the medical department had been rather lax over recent vaccinations – a charge vigorously denied by the Deputy Governor. Certainly, the government and missions carried out extensive public vaccination programmes: between 1911 and 1913 over 380,000 individual vaccinations were reported. The Principal Medical Officers (PMOs) believed that the vaccination campaigns had effectively eradicated smallpox. However, Rennick has pointed out more recently that the reduction may have been due to changes in smallpox epidemiology, and that the statistics may have been incorrect, as their compilation was unreliable.[43]

From this emerging picture, it is clear that the contributions of missions were crucial to the implementation of the vaccination campaigns: missions provided skilled personnel and enabled colonial medical services to reach districts where there was no official presence. Furthermore, in established areas the missionaries and their African associates had intimate knowledge of local conditions and were known by the local population. For the government, vaccination campaigns were cost-effective: in 1913, the PMO reported that the medical department had spent the relatively meagre sum of £200 to pay 'Native Vaccinators' and a further £100 for the lymph supply.[44]

For missionaries, cooperation with the government generated goodwill. They received more resources and the backing of the colonial state to carry out large-scale vaccinations, which in turn extended the medical missions' evangelistic reach. It is evident that the missions used vaccination campaigns for their own religious ends. For example, at Bandawe station in 1900, one Livingstonia evangelist and medical assistant preached to the people who had gathered to be vaccinated, emphasising through the power of analogy that Christianity offered protection against 'the disease of sin in the heart'.[45] The early vaccinators were mostly mission-educated men; probably many of them were also Christian teachers, church elders and evangelists. It is possible that they carried out evangelisation whilst employed by the government. Many vaccinators worked in remote districts without European supervision.[46] In 1902, Laws reported to PMO Hearsey that he had sent two Livingstonia 'lads' to carry out vaccinations amongst the Senga. In 1906, Hearsey sent lymph to all eight Livingstonia doctors. Livingstonia doctors in Northern Rhodesia also took part in vaccination campaigns.[47] In Malawi, government and mission cooperation in vaccination continued at least into the 1940s.[48]

Some similarities in this spirit of informal cooperation can be seen in approaches to sleeping sickness epidemics. In 1907, James Chisholm (Livingstonia) in Mwenzo, North Rhodesia examined a blood sample taken from a dying patient who had arrived from the Belgian Congo. Chisholm diagnosed a case of sleeping sickness, which was to become a major threat to the British administrations in both Nyasaland and Northern Rhodesia.[49] The geographical location of Livingstonia stations in the border region put mission doctors in an important position in early colonial responses to sleeping sickness. Although it did not become a major concern for the UMCA,[50] initial campaigns against sleeping sickness also involved the Blantyre Mission and the Dutch Reformed Church Mission.[51]

The spread of sleeping sickness to British Central African territories had been feared for some time before Chisholm's diagnosis, not least because in Uganda the disease had caused hundreds of thousands of deaths in the epidemic that ravaged the Lake Victoria region between 1901 and 1905. In December 1906, Laws had informed PMO Hearsey of the presence of sleeping sickness and tsetse fly in the Congo.[52] George Prentice, then stationed at Kasungu, became a key Livingstonia doctor in the debates about preventative measures. In 1907, having been asked to temporarily take on the role of MO at Fort Jameson in Northern Rhodesia, Prentice was in no doubt that the missions and government had to join forces.[53] The Nyasaland medical department established an outpost for inspecting travellers from potentially infected regions in 1907. In 1909, Hardy of the Colonial Medical Service died of sleeping sickness, and fears of an epidemic prompted the additional recruitment of MOs as well as the establishment of a Sleeping Sickness Commission in 1911 (headed by Sir David Bruce) to investigate the threat in detail.[54]

The colonial government attempted to establish strict movement restrictions within the perceived sleeping sickness zones and to quarantine and inspect every suspected disease carrier. Those suspected of infection were to be sent to isolation camps. The implementation of these practical procedures relied upon missionary doctors to carry out inspections. Perhaps ironically, particular attention was paid to members of the Livingstonia mission community, which was viewed as harbouring a suspiciously mobile population of teachers, evangelists and pupils who frequently travelled over the border zone into the infected areas. Some of the first confirmed victims of sleeping sickness were mission teachers.[55]

At first it was assumed that raised cervical glands were a sign of possible infection, with both missionaries and colonial doctors routinely examining tens of thousands of Africans by palpating their glands. By 1908 this technique had been deemed unreliable: the majority of those with enlarged glands were not infected and thus could be wrongly isolated. Gland puncture provided a more reliable diagnostic tool, but the technique was feared and resented. Initially, as Rennick notes, gland palpation focused on mission pupils and African workers employed by Europeans. As fears of an epidemic grew, the government resorted to greater force in carrying out sleeping sickness examinations, with MOs sometimes reinforced by armed police.[56] But although such forcible examples of procuring a diagnosis were associated with the government medical service, collaboration still very much lay at the heart of successful sleeping sickness eradication initiatives. The government medical department regularly called upon mission doctors to palpate and puncture the glands of their patients, microscopically inspect blood specimens and send infected individuals to isolation camps. The acting PMO, Norris, a former Blantyre doctor, articulated the reliance on medical missionaries when he declared them as the personnel who were generally in 'the best position to undertake gland palpitation and puncture'.[57] The use of medical missionaries was all the more expedient, given that missionary doctors were believed to be more trusted than those in the employment of the government, at least by those in mission communities.

By 1910, George Prentice of the Livingstonia Mission had become a vocal critic of government tsetse and sleeping sickness policies. For Prentice, tsetse and consequently sleeping sickness depended 'entirely upon the presence of big game', which had increased as a result of government policies of game protection that had deprived Africans of their hunting rights. In his annual report for 1910, Prentice stated that each victim of sleeping sickness, or 'tsetse fever', was 'a martyr to our policy of game protection', which had also robbed the people of their lawful food supply. He was highly critical of the way the administration had forcibly removed Africans from areas that were seen as potential sleeping sickness danger zones. Whilst Prentice believed that game, tsetse and the local populations could not safely inhabit the same area, he argued that the government had foolishly 'moved the people and left the game' in at least one area. Furthermore, he held that amongst the medical profession in the Protectorate, only government doctors supported this highly erroneous official policy. In his call for reform, Prentice called upon Scottish churches to press for progressive policies against tsetse that would include the restoration of hunting rights and the establishment of a cotton industry in Central Nyasaland. Such agricultural expansion, he argued, would also provide labour for those who had been forced to migrate. Whilst Prentice believed that the Protectorate was facing 'the biggest crisis this country has ever known', he clearly also believed that harnessing missionary support was vital to persuade colonial MOs to take up the measures that he felt would prevent any new outbreak from reaching epidemic proportions.[58]

The debate that ensued is indicative. Prentice's views were supported by Alexander Hetherwick, head of Blantyre, who became the spokesman for the united Scottish missionaries in Scotland and held a position in the Legislative Council in Zomba. Ideas about game destruction were fiercely opposed by Governor Alfred Sharpe, however. In Britain, the Scottish churches' deputation managed to secure a Sleeping

Sickness Commission in 1911, and one game reserve (Elephant Marsh) was abolished. Whilst Prentice was invited to provide medical facts for the Scottish churches, he was not asked to speak in Britain, allegedly because of his poor oratory skills.[59]

The reasons for the lack of a coordinated response seem clear. Sleeping sickness regulations, inspections and isolation measures that often resembled military campaigns provoked strong resentment from local societies. They also considerably hampered the other work of the Livingstonia missionaries.[60] In the end, sleeping sickness did not materialise in Malawi to the extent that had been feared. At the outbreak of the First World War, the Sleeping Sickness Commission was withdrawn and the medical department was prepared instead for military duty. Prentice's extensive ecological and economic anti-tsetse initiatives were not adopted, although short-lived free-shooting zones were set up in 1915, which were alleged to have merely scattered the big game and spread the tsetse further.[61]

The story of plague responses in colonial Malawi reveals particularly interesting examples of cooperation over health issues. In December 1916, Saulos Nyirenda and Yafet Gondwe, two Livingstonia graduates and church elders from Mchenga village near Karonga, sent the following telegraph to Dr Innes of the mission: 'We are dying [in] our village investigate come immediately.' Innes went to Mchenga, where at least three children of Christian families had died suddenly. On analysing samples, he identified a plague bacillus. The administration then sent an MO, who confirmed the diagnosis in March 1917. A large-scale plague emergency ensued, comprising travel restrictions and a major rat-destruction campaign.[62]

Mission-educated African Christians also played an important role in informing villagers about anti-plague measures and orders. During the initial plague panic, the Livingstonia doctors were closest to the epidemic and advised concerned colonial officials. Laws assured the Resident at Karonga, for example, that steaming all letters was an unnecessary measure and instead advocated the strict control of all traffic over the Rukuru river.[63] The spirit of advice and cooperation continued and in 1919 Laws sent all the kittens from the Livingstonia headquarters for rat-hunting duty in the threatened villages.[64]

The plague alert resulted in considerable travel restrictions in the North and West Nyasa Districts and medical certificates for both European and African travellers continued to be required for years after the initial outbreak. Livingstonia doctors Laws and Innes undertook examinations and certifications in 1917 and 1918.[65] However, by early 1919, with the arrival of a government MO in Karonga, the examinations were to become the preserve of MO Arbuckle. Unsurprisingly, this decision prompted sharp criticism from Laws, who, robbed of his former authority, bluntly asked why the mission doctors should now be considered 'less competent' to carry out examinations and whether in the possible absence of Dr Arbuckle all monitoring of traffic in the districts would grind to a halt.[66]

This exchange over plague examinations highlights one area of professional contestation between colonial and missionary doctors: the question of competence and authority. Whilst the government responded quickly to missionary alerts in both sleeping sickness and plague cases, frequently it can be seen that the MOs wanted to confirm the diagnoses themselves. This, I suggest, has to be seen in the context of the development of a distinct colonial medical elite with specialist training in tropical medicine. By the early 1900s, British MOs posted to the tropics were increasingly trained at the London and Liverpool schools of tropical medicine. A key element in their training was laboratory work; particularly carrying out microscopic investigations to identify disease-causing agents.[67] This emergence of specialised elite experts in tropical medicine from the metropole contributed to questioning of and increasing conflict with local experts in the colonies, such as medical missionaries, who, especially in the early years of the century, tended to rely on authority gained through prolonged residency in the same locality. Laws was a prime example of this older kind of expert on health. However, this conflict should not be over-emphasised. It should also be noted that in Malawi the younger generation of missionary doctors, including Chisholm and Prentice, also took specialist tropical medicine courses in Britain and obtained qualifications to carry out laboratory research in Africa.[68]

As the Nyasaland colonial medical service began to extend into areas where previously missions had dominated Western medicine and public health, contests over authority occurred, as highlighted by the debate over plague rules and the substitution of Arbuckle for Laws. In the absence of government doctors from Karonga and in the context of the war, there was no difficulty in granting Livingstonia missionaries authority to issue travel certificates on public health grounds, but as the situation began to normalise in 1919, Arbuckle seems to have wanted to assert his authority as a government MO by assuming sole responsibility for medical certification.

Leprosy collaboration in the interwar era

As elsewhere in the British Empire, leprosy relief in Malawi brought government and missions together in formal collaboration in the interwar period. The government subsidised the treatment of leprosy patients through modest sums and medicinal provision, while in Nyasaland the UMCA pioneered the treatment of leprosy patients. In the 1920s, the Scottish missions, Seventh Day Adventists and White Fathers also established leprosy settlements or treatment centres.[69] In 1934, the government provided an annual sum of £900 to cover all mission leprosy work, plus £100 towards leprosy and hookworm drugs. Despite an admission of the inadequacy of this subsidy, it remained roughly the same into the 1940s. By 1940, about 600 leprosy patients, mostly men, were said to be resident in mission settlements.[70]

From 1927 onwards, the Nyasaland Medical Department began to scrutinise the use of leprosy grants. The DMS called into question the grant for the UMCA's Likoma leprosy settlement, on the grounds that most of its patients came from Portuguese territory. In the late 1930s the medical department was, in Good's words, 'staking out its professional and "turf" positions'. Whilst admitting the value of mission services for leprosy patients, medical services now sought the power to inspect mission facilities as required and to authorise grant reductions if 'approved standards' were not met.[71]

It has been noted that leprosy relief was specially treated in the modern British Empire, as it largely remained an uncontested area, primarily regarded as being in the preserve of missionary medicine. Colonial medical services were willing to provide funds for leprosy care to missions, and missions willingly accepted responsibility, making reference to the spiritual tradition surrounding the care of lepers that went back to Christ. Thus, for an arguably rather small outlay, government medical services in Malawi were able to rid themselves of responsibility for a major disease. In 1927 the government estimated that there were about 6,000 leprosy patients in the Protectorate, most of them cared for by missions, often at the expense of other medical work. The rationale seems clear: for the missions, leprosy collaboration was a means of demonstrating their value to, and maintaining good relations with, both the medical department specifically and the colonial government more generally.[72] Leprosy was not a high-profile tropical disease, nor was it a major threat to the colonial administration, but its treatment required long-term commitment and personnel – thus, given its low public profile, the medical services were happy to 'subcontract' its treatment to the missions.

Exchanges of material and information

Tracing the exchange of medicines also provides insight into informal collaborative trends between missions and the government medical department. As noted above, vaccine lymph, despite its unreliability, was one of the more successful materials exchanged by government and missionary doctors, but this was just one of the many *materia medica* exchanged. In 1918, as the influenza pandemic spread to South-Central Africa, MOs in Northern Rhodesia sent serum for influenza 'inoculation' to missionaries at Chitambo.[73] In the interwar era, the Nyasaland Medical Department supplied some missions with medicines for the treatment of yaws, bilharzia and hookworm, as well as leprosy. In 1933, leprosy drugs for the UMCA included Moogrol and Chaulmoogra oils, trichloroacetic acid and potassium iodide.[74]

The sharing of information and knowledge was also important in campaigns against epidemic disease, when not only missionaries, but also mission-educated Africans played a significant part in reporting disease and acting as intermediaries for government instructions. Similarly, the colonial doctors turned to their mission colleagues for information on the African population, prevalence of disease or symptoms. Thus the mission doctors played a part in the construction of a colonial medical discourse: they charted, assessed and measured health, illness and susceptibility to disease, often in areas of the Protectorate where few government doctors were posted.[75] On the basis of his long experience and status, Laws became a key informant for the government on African infant mortality, birth rate and perceived changes in population during his fifty-year period in Malawi.[76]

Missionary doctors and nurses also informed the authorities about cases of violence and suspected poisonings that came to their attention. However, medico-legal cooperation could be problematic. In the 1910s, the government wanted to enlist mission doctors to carry out post-mortem examinations where administration doctors were not available. Whilst Laws was keen to assist the authorities whenever possible, he strongly rejected any suggestion that mission doctors should be forced to carry out post-mortem examinations and to actually exhume the bodies (practices that were viewed with suspicion by the majority of the African population). He was reassured by MO Hugh Stannus that in cases of suspected foul play, corpses would be delivered to investigating doctors – both government and missionary.[77]

Medical education and African medical staff

Unlike European medical staff, there was considerable mobility from missions to government medical service among African medical assistants, orderlies and probably nurses. These were the crucial 'medical middles' who enabled the expansion of both missionary and colonial medicine, and missions dominated medical training and education at least until the Second World War.

In early colonial Malawi, the missions ran some of the most ambitious medical training schemes in Anglophone Africa, and for a while the Scottish missions in particular trained African medical middles for employment beyond the Protectorate. The more advanced Hospital Assistant training in Blantyre and Livingstonia took three or four years to complete.[78] Robert Laws was especially active in this area. As a member of the Legislative Council between 1913 and 1916, Laws wanted to create a Christian, mission-trained medical profession, first for assistants, and later also for nurses and midwives. By the First World War, the three British missions all ran some form of formal medical training scheme, and issued certificates to their graduates. By 1926, the most highly trained Hospital Assistants were registered by the government; however, most African medical staff members were not.[79]

In contrast to this relatively organised provision, before the 1920s, the government undertook practically no formal training of subsidiary medical staff, and even in the interwar period its programmes were modest in comparison to those run by the three leading British missions. Despite their lack of early tangible success, the colonial medical services clearly sought to develop training programmes in Zomba, as is apparent from PMO Hearsey's medical report for 1919.[80] By 1923 Hearsey was able to report that the majority of state rural dispensaries were run by government-trained dispensers, although their period of training was well short of the three or four years required by the missions.[81] Significantly, however, all government dispensers were former mission pupils. Furthermore, their training in Zomba was largely undertaken by senior African staff (including Thomas Cheonga and Daniel Gondwe in 1928), all of whom were mission-trained men.[82]

In 1936, the government opened its Medical Training School in Zomba. It offered courses for medical dressers, nurses and midwives, as well as laboratory assistants and sanitary inspectors. However, the Hospital Assistants seem to have been still exclusively mission trained. The African staff employed by the government increased from 3 hospital assistants and 132 medical dressers in 1927 to 16 Hospital Assistants and 215 dressers in 1937.[83]

African medical middles, especially the elite Hospital Assistants, therefore should be seen as constituting a significant connecting group between missionary and colonial medicine. Some middles moved directly from mission training into government service, others worked for long periods for the missions before taking up government employment. For example, Fred Nyirenda, a Livingstonia medical graduate, worked for Livingstonia for some years before being seconded into government service during the plague emergency. It appears that Nyirenda was not at first formally recruited, but 'on loan' from the mission.[84] However, he was to become a key worker when the government hospital in Karonga was permanently established. In 1927, upon the recommendation of the DMS, Nyirenda was registered as a 'Native Hospital Assistant' under the new Medical Practitioners Ordinance.[85] By 1939 he had become a first-grade Hospital Assistant. At that point, the medical department employed one senior, nine first-grade and six junior Hospital Assistants.[86]

Some middles moved across East Africa, including Dan Ngurube, one of the most highly trained Hospital Assistant graduates of Livingstonia. Ngurube graduated in 1933, in 1939 was promoted to Senior Hospital Assistant, first grade, and was at the top of African staff scale in the Nyasaland Medical Department. Later, Ngurube moved to the government medical department in Tanganyika.[87]

For some, the move into government service was precipitated by conflict with the mission. Daniel Gondwe, the first formally trained hospital assistant of Livingstonia, lost his position because of mission objections to his polygamous marriage in the late 1910s. Discussing the case in 1920, Laws maintained that, as a polygamist, Gondwe had become permanently 'unstable'. The government had no such qualms, however: by 1924 Gondwe was listed as one of three African Hospital Assistants in the medical department.[88]

Missionaries wanted to keep African medical middles under control and supervision, and made this clear to the government.[89] For its part, the colonial medical department did not see the mission domination of subordinate medical education as particularly problematic and was keen to employ mission-educated medical staff. The Nyasaland Medical Department offered employment for only some mission graduates. In addition to British and African staff, the government employed Indian Sub-Assistant Surgeons (SAS): their rank was between MOs and hospital assistants, and they occupied an important middle position that otherwise might have been filled by the elite of African middles. Indeed, Laws seems to have hoped that African hospital assistants would eventually replace SASs. Practicalities hindered his ambitions, however, as by the early 1930s the most advanced medical courses at Livingstonia had to be scaled down and the supply of highly trained medical middles began to decline. When the last group of Livingstonia assistants graduated in 1933, their examination and registration by the state was a well-established process. They were examined in physiology, anatomy, hygiene and pharmacology, and the DMS noted that they were the best group that had been examined to date. After 1933, higher medical training for Africans was concentrated at the Blantyre Mission main hospital.[90]

Government service offered higher salaries to African medical middles than the financially struggling missions of the 1920s could.

There is evidence that Malawian graduates had a good reputation and that they were regularly sought after by other British administrations: notably Tanganyika and the Rhodesias. The PMO of Tanganyika, for example, contacted Laws in 1925 and asked for sixteen new medical workers. Laws replied that Livingstonia needed the sanction of the Nyasaland government to be able to formally train staff for other British territories and that it could not immediately provide such numbers.[91] Although these types of requests sometimes contained an offer to subsidise the training of any staff thus supplied, this was not always the case. In 1924 Laws noted dryly that the PMO in Northern Rhodesia expected rather too much in anticipating the provision of trained assistants for free.[92] In the interwar era, Tanganyika, the Rhodesias and South Africa were able to provide more favourable rates of pay to Malawian assistants. In this competitive environment the Nyasaland medical services, with lower salaries and few positions, were able to hire only some mission graduates.[93]

By the Second World War, the training of African nurses and mid-wives had become a priority for both the missions and the colonial medical services. The mission midwifery training undertaken at Blantyre, Livingstonia and Mlanda (Dutch Reformed Church) was recognised by the medical service.[94] The ambitious new DMS, Dr De Boer, argued that the medical department needed reorganisation, more European and African staff and other resources. He clearly wanted to take over the medical education of African male assistants and order-lies from the missions. By 1940, the government offered free medical training in Zomba (by contrast, Blantyre charged its pupils), which the Scottish missionaries regarded as a serious threat.[95] De Boer planned to gradually replace the Indian SASs with African Hospital Assistants, who were cheaper agents: in 1939 the salary of one SAS (£236) covered the wages of three Hospital Assistants.[96] Although de Boer's sugges-tions for the wide-ranging reform of the medical services were generally welcomed by the authorities in London and Zomba, after war broke out it became clear that the necessary resources would not be forthcoming, and the scheme never was to fulfil his ambitious intentions.[97]

Private critiques, muted conflicts

On the surface, early twentieth-century mission–government relations on issues of medicine and health appear relatively untroubled. Conflict was more apparent in other areas of policy, such as Blantyre missionar-ies' critique of Johnston's administration, or the debate about mission education in the aftermath of the Chilembwe Rising in 1915. Prentice's attack on the government's sleeping sickness policies was an example of a rare public outburst by a missionary physician. More usually, missionary criticism of government activities remained private, as the correspondence of Laws attests.

The First World War put particular pressure on mission–government cooperation. In 1917, Laws strongly criticised the administration for failing to provide a single MO for civilian duty and for absorbing mission doctors into a large medical department for the small armed force. In a similar vein, after the government and Livingstonia disagreed over payment of mission doctors' services for plague duty, Laws lambasted the administration for not valuing the services of mission doctors. Perhaps more important than money, professional respect was at stake. Furthermore, Laws questioned the quality of treatment provided to Africans in colonial military service during the war. Livingstonia hospital had received several gravely ill Africans who were discharged from service and practically left to die. For those sick African carriers who made it to the mission hospital, the government offered to pay for a maximum stay of fourteen days as an in-patient, or £1 1s. In a letter to the Chief Secretary, Laws described how carriers were suffering from dysentery, chronic ulcers and hunger, and pointed out that a question put to the House of Commons on the subject 'would be an exceedingly awkward one for the Government here to answer'.[98] However, publicly, Livingstonia, which had fully cooperated with the recruitment of carriers for war service, remained silent.[99]

In 1940, when the British missions were alarmed by the planned reorganisation of the Nyasaland medical services by DMS De Boer, they appealed directly to the authorities in London for support. Scottish missions, in particular, feared that the government would monopolise medicine and medical education in Nyasaland and sought reassurance that there was still room for medical missions in the country. The complaints were expressed semi-officially. Mapping this process of rather subtle appeal and complaint is revealing of the caution that clearly underscored fragile interrelations between missions and state. The Church of Scotland missionaries contacted H.M. Grace, the chairman of the Conference of Missionary Societies in Great Britain, who informed the Colonial Office that the relations between the DMS and Livingstonia in particular were 'very unsatisfactory' and that there was 'a spirit of competition by Government', which made complementary medical policy very difficult.[100] Grace then had an interview with Sir Jameson at the Colonial Office, from which he left satisfied with the friendly discussions they had undertaken on the subject. In a subsequent note, Grace emphasised that he had been contacted by four important societies in Nyasaland that had had difficulties with the DMS, but all their communications had been confidential.[101]

[56]

The precise details of the mission complaints remain obscure. However, it is clear that the missionaries thought that the new government medical training programme at Zomba, which offered free education and a subsistence allowance, undercut mission medical education at Blantyre. At this stage, Blantyre charged its medical students £5 per year, and its student numbers had been halved. Missionaries stated that they had not been officially informed about the Zomba training centre at all and that there had been no discussion of the co-existence of the two institutions. In the meeting at the Colonial Office, Jameson believed that missions and government could find a workable division of labour, ideally one that allowed missions to focus on the training of public health nurses and midwives, for example.[102]

In this contest, missions and medical service were competing above all about African 'boys' as medical students. De Boer was willing to let missions train nurses, but wanted the training of men in government hands. Jameson believed that on financial grounds it was clear that the missions could not carry out the most advanced training.[103] With the benefit of hindsight it can be seen that this contest was ultimately nothing more than a storm in a teacup: De Boer's ambitious reform plans had to be shelved during the war. However, it still serves as an illustrative example that the struggle over Western medicine in Malawi was turning towards the medical services' favour. Whilst the medical services were under-resourced, by 1940 the medical missions were weak and unable to maintain a monopoly in Blantyre. De Boer found that the Blantyre mission hospital could not serve as a site for the planned government hospitals for Europeans, Africans and Asians, as its buildings 'had nearly served their period of usefulness'. However, De Boer acknowledged that the medical services had no funds or desire to expand into remote areas that were adequately served by missions. The growing town of Blantyre, in turn, had sufficient African population to justify both government and mission hospitals.[104] The 1940 conflict remained largely obscure even for some of those involved. Jameson confessed that after the friendly talk with Grace, he still did not 'know the ins and outs of this matter at all' and asked de Boer for further, unofficial information.[105] It seems clear in practice that to no small degree, and despite a veneer of collaboration, competition, professional jealousy and lack of contact prohibited extensive cooperation.

Conclusion

Colonial medical services and British missions in Malawi exchanged and shared information, materials and personnel. Mission-educated African medical middles provided a crucial skilled workforce for the expanding medical department, and material exchanges were regularly undertaken, albeit on an *ad hoc* rather than formal basis. Yet, despite these examples of fluidity between the two groups, they strongly retained their distinct boundaries. Geography determined mission–government relations in medicine and healthcare. The UMCA in its 'steamer parish' across Lake Malawi and Livingstonia in the north were in more remote and thus independent positions. As their network of stations, congregations and African and European medical staff extended far beyond the government's presence, collaboration with these missions enabled the administration to reach local societies. In the Shire Highlands, where colonial and missionary medicine overlapped, a division of labour was cost-effective: the mission concentrated on Blantyre and African patients, the Colonial Service on Zomba and government employees. Colonial medicine in Malawi focused more on men, particularly able-bodied government workers, soldiers and labourers. Missions treated more women, children, elderly patients (cataract operations were a particular strength of mission surgery in the early 1900s) and leprosy patients.

Missions mediated knowledge, practices and materials between the fragile colonial state and African societies. They informed the administration of local disease conditions, people's health and their views on improvement. They also helped to ensure the enactment of government regulations, orders and advice regarding illness and health, and in turn strove to influence government decision making in these fields. In the early period, some missionaries exerted quasi-official authority in enforcing health regulations, thus becoming *de facto* MOs. However, as colonial medical services in Nyasaland strengthened in the 1920s, the medical department took a more critical attitude towards medical missions and mission doctors, and increasingly insisted upon its hegemony over medical and public health policy, authority and practice.

By the Second World War, the medical department's professional and administrative ambition to have the final say on all publicly funded medical and health practice was most apparent in leprosy collaboration as well as in competing claims to have the monopoly in African medical education. With hindsight, if British missions and the government medical department had pooled their resources, they could have established a strong medical school for the Protectorate, but such extensive collaboration seems not to have been on the agenda, either for missions or for the government – both of whom wanted control over Africans trained in medicine and nursing in their respective institutions. For missionaries, such a wish must have had its roots in attempts to exert religious control and moral scrutiny. For the colonial

MOs, secular professional demands for administrative hegemony probably prevented more extensive cooperation. In the end, the African population, the government and the missions were all left without an adequate number of African medical staff.

Finally, the 1940 conflict surrounding De Boer's reforms highlighted how the British missions, with their representatives in Edinburgh and London, could make their cases and take their complaints to the higher echelons of the Colonial Service, but these exchanges left only faint traces in official records. On the surface, the British missions and colonial administration seemed unified in their championing of Western medicine and public health, but underneath there were significant fractures in their cooperation.

This study of collaboration, connections and conflicts between missions and the Colonial Medical Service reminds us that Western medicine in the colonial world was not monolithic or marked by simple dualism between state and churches or secular and spiritual agents. Medical practice, practitioners, knowledge and materials were constituted, transferred and connected in complex imperial networks that included MOs, missionary physicians and various medical middles. Both cooperation and conflicts occurred within these networks, and the fuller understanding of colonial medicine in both local and imperial contexts requires sensitivity to these informal agents, exchanges and connections.

Acknowledgements

I would like to thank Anna Greenwood, Ryan Johnson and Liz Eastcott for their invaluable help in improving this chapter (all omissions or errors are naturally my own). The research has been made possible thanks to funding from the Academy of Finland (project no. 121514) and the Department of History and Ethnology, University of Jyväskylä.

Notes

1   Megan Vaughan, *Curing Their Ills: Colonial Power and African Illness*, Cambridge, Polity Press, 1991, p. 56
2   Charles Good, *The Steamer Parish: The Rise and Fall of Missionary Medicine on an African Frontier*, London, University of Chicago Press, 2004, p. 278
3   For an overview of the history of Western medicine in Malawi, see Michael King and Elspeth King, *The Story of Medicine and Disease in Malawi: The 150 Years Since Livingstone*, Blantyre, The Montfort Press, 1997. On missionary medicine, see Good, *The Steamer Parish*; Markku Hokkanen, *Medicine and Scottish Missionaries in the Northern Malawi Region: Quests for Health in a Colonial Society*, Lewiston, The Edwin Mellen Press, 2007; Agnes Rennick, 'Church and Medicine: The Role of Medical Missionaries in Malawi 1875–1914', unpublished PhD thesis, University of Stirling, 2003; Vaughan, *Curing Their Ills*. On Colonial

Medical Service, see Colin Baker, 'The Government Medical Service in Malawi', *Medical History*, 20, 3, 1976, pp. 296–311

4   Vaughan, *Curing Their Ills*; Rennick, 'Church and Medicine'; Hokkanen, *Medicine and Scottish Missionaries*
5   There were other Catholic and Protestant missions in Malawi practising medicine, but in the colonial period the three main British missions were predominant
6   Baker, 'The Government Medical Service'
7   Good, *The Steamer Parish*
8   Michael Worboys, 'The Colonial World as Mission and Mandate: Leprosy and Empire, 1900–1940', *Osiris*, 15, 2000, pp. 207–18
9   For Livingstonia, see John McCracken, *Politics and Christianity in Malawi: The Impact of the Livingstonia Mission in the Northern Province*, Blantyre, CLAIM, 2000; Hokkanen, *Medicine and Scottish Missionaries*
10 Good, *The Steamer Parish*; Rennick, 'Church and Medicine'
11 Rennick, 'Church and Medicine', p. 37; McCracken, *Politics and Christianity*, pp. 147–9, 212; Hokkanen, *Medicine and Scottish Missionaries*, pp. 73–4, 77–8, 156
12 Ronald Oliver, *The Missionary Factor in East Africa*, London, Longmans, 1952, pp. 109–28; Colin Baker, 'The Development of the Administration to 1897', in Bridglal Pachai (ed.), *The Early History of Malawi*, London, Northwestern University Press, 1972
13 Rennick, 'Church and Medicine', p. 46; Andrew C. Ross, *Blantyre Mission and the Making of Modern Malawi*, Blantyre, CLAIM, 1996
14 McCracken, *Politics and Christianity*, pp. 147–9
15 Baker, 'The Government Medical Service', pp. 296–8; King and King, *The Story of Medicine*, pp. 90, 103
16 Rennick, 'Church and Medicine', p. 317
17 Rennick, 'Church and Medicine', pp. 328–30
18 The National Archives, UK (TNA) CO/626/19 Nyasaland Protectorate Administration Reports 1939, Annual Report of the Social and Economic Progress of the People of Nyasaland for the Year 1939, p. 7; Nyasaland Protectorate, *Annual Medical Report for 1914*, Zomba, 1915; Nyasaland Protectorate, *Annual Medical Report for 1928*, Zomba, 1929
19 Good, *The Steamer Parish*; Hokkanen, *Medicine and Scottish Missionaries*; Rennick, 'Church and Medicine'
20 Rennick, 'Church and Medicine', pp. 338–9
21 Rennick, 'Church and Medicine', p. 338; Hokkanen, *Medicine and Scottish Missionaries*
22 Rennick, 'Church and Medicine', pp. 124–6, 232–8
23 Vaughan, *Curing Their Ills*, pp. 100–1, 107–10; Megan Vaughan, 'Idioms of Madness: Zomba Lunatic Asylum, Nyasaland, in the Colonial Period', *Journal of Southern African Studies*, 9, 2, 1983, pp. 218–38, at 218–21
24 Baker, 'The Government Medical Service', pp. 301–4
25 TNA CO/626/19 Nyasaland Protectorate Administration Reports 1939, Annual Report of the Social and Economic Progress of the People of Nyasaland for the Year 1939, p. 4
26 TNA CO/626/5, Nyasaland Protectorate Proceedings (Minutes) of the Executive Council 1920–1925, Minutes of the Executive Council, 18 December 1923
27 Malawi National Archives (MNA) 47/LIM/1/24 Letterbook of Laws, 1924–1925, letters 266 and 310, Laws to Fraser, 3 and 18 March 1925
28 Vaughan, *Curing Their Ills*, p. 23
29 For the benefits of a colonial medical career see Anna Crozier, *Practising Colonial Medicine: The Colonial Medical Service in East Africa*, London, I.B. Tauris, 2007, pp. 46–71
30 Hokkanen, *Medicine and Scottish Missionaries*, pp. 365–6
31 Rennick, 'Church and Medicine', pp. 151, 238–9
32 TNA CO/525/184/14, De Boer to Chief Secretary, 31 July 1940

33 Baker, 'The Government Medical Service', p. 307; The Registration of Medical Practitioners Ordinance, No. 9 of 1906, [? *British Central Africa Gazette*, 1906]

34 TNA CO/626/8, Nyasaland Executive Council Minutes, 1926–1930, Minutes of the Executive Council, 8 September 1927; King and King, *The Story of Medicine*, pp. 136–7. For the rising, see George Shepperson and Thomas Price, *Independent African*, Edinburgh, Edinburgh University Press, 1958; John McCracken, *A History of Malawi*, Woodbridge, James Currey, 2012, pp. 127–46

35 TNA CO/525/184/14, De Boer to Chief Secretary, 31 July 1940

36 Vaughan, *Curing Their Ills*, p. 23

37 John Lwanda, 'Politics, Culture and Medicine in Malawi: Historical Continuities and Ruptures with Special Reference to HIV/AIDS', unpublished PhD thesis, University of Edinburgh, 2002, p. 76

38 Good, *The Steamer Parish*, pp. 238–40; Eugenia W. Herbert, 'Smallpox Inoculation in Africa', *Journal of African History*, 16, 4, 1975, pp. 539–59; Lwanda, 'Politics, Culture and Medicine', pp. 65–7

39 Hokkanen, *Medicine and Scottish Missionaries*, p. 146; Rennick, 'Church and Medicine', p. 297

40 Hokkanen, *Medicine and Scottish Missionaries*, pp. 146, 298; Rennick, 'Church and Medicine', p. 302

41 Rennick, 'Church and Medicine', pp. 297–300

42 Good, *The Steamer Parish*, p. 274

43 Rennick, 'Church and Medicine', pp. 301–2; TNA CO/626/6, Nyasaland Protectorate Legislative Council Minutes, 1908–1925, Summary of the Proceedings of the Legislative Council of Nyasaland, 2nd session, 5 to 7 November 1908

44 *Annual Medical Report*, 31 December 1913, quoted in Rennick, 'Church and Medicine', p. 301

45 *Free Church of Scotland Monthly Record*, January 1901, pp. 17–19; Hokkanen, *Medicine and Scottish Missionaries*, pp. 353–4

46 Rennick, 'Church and Medicine', p. 302

47 MNA 47/LIM/1/1/9, Overtoun Institution Letterbook 1906–1908, letters 172 and 17, Laws to Hearsey, 2 December 1906, enclosure from Laws to Hearsey, no date; Hokkanen, *Medicine and Scottish Missionaries*, p. 482

48 Good, *The Steamer Parish*, pp. 380–2

49 Hokkanen, *Medicine and Scottish Missionaries*, pp. 484–6

50 Good, *The Steamer Parish*, p. 251

51 Rennick, 'Church and Medicine', pp. 307–10

52 MNA 47/LIM/1/1/9, Overtoun Institution Letterbook 1906–1908, letters 172 and 17, Laws to Hearsey, 2 December 1906

53 National Library of Scotland, Edinburgh (NLS) Acc/7548/D71, Letters to the Livingstonia Sub-Committee 1907, p. 71, Prentice, 9 May 1907

54 Baker, 'The Government Medical Service', pp. 298–9

55 *The Livingstonia News*, October 1909, p. 65; Nyasaland Protectorate, *Report of Commissioner for 1912–1913*, Cmd. 7050, London, 1913, pp. 22–3; Hokkanen, *Medicine and Scottish Missionaries*, p. 485

56 Rennick, 'Church and Medicine', pp. 308–10

57 MNA 50/BMC/2/1/96, Norris to Hetherwick, 2 December 1908, quoted in Rennick, 'Church and Medicine', p. 310

58 *Annual Report of the Livingstonia Mission for 1910*, Glasgow, 1911, pp. 27–9

59 Rennick, 'Church and Medicine', pp. 312–6

60 Hokkanen, *Medicine and Scottish Missionaries*, p. 486

61 Baker, 'The Government Medical Service', p. 300; Good, *The Steamer Parish*, pp. 250–1; Hokkanen, *Medicine and Scottish Missionaries*, p. 486; John McCracken, 'Experts and Expertise in Colonial Malawi', *African Affairs*, 81, 1982, pp. 101–16, at p. 107. For a comparable case of co-operation during the plague emergency in Accra, see Ryan Johnson, '*Mantsemei*, Interpreters and the Successful Eradication of Plague: The 1908 Plague Epidemic in Colonial Accra', in Ryan Johnson and Amna

Khalid (eds.), *Public Health in the British Empire: Intermediaries, Subordinates, and the Practice of Public Health, 1850–1960*, New York, Routledge, 2012

62 MNA 47/LIM/1/1/17, Laws to Resident, Karonga, 18 December 1916; Hokkanen, *Medicine and Scottish Missionaries*, pp. 488–9

63 MNA 47/LIM/1/1/17, letters 853 and 906, Laws to MacDonald, 19 February and 14 March 1917; Hokkanen, *Medicine and Scottish Missionaries*, pp. 489–90

64 MNA 47/LIM/1/19, Overtoun Institution Letterbook 1919–1921, letter 292, Laws to Hearsey, 16 October 1919. On rat eradication campaigns, see Vaughan, *Curing Their Ills*, pp. 39–43

65 Hokkanen, *Medicine and Scottish Missionaries*, pp. 488–92

66 MNA 47/LIM/1/1/19, Overtoun Institution Letterbook 1919–1921, letter 79, Laws to Arbuckle, 21 May 1919

67 Deborah Neill, *Networks in Tropical Medicine: Internationalism, Colonialism, and the Rise of a Medical Speciality 1890–1930*, Stanford, Stanford University Press, 2012, pp. 60–5

68 Hokkanen, *Medicine and Scottish Missionaries*

69 Good, *The Steamer Parish*, pp. 337–9; Worboys, 'The Colonial World'

70 Good, *The Steamer Parish*, pp. 337–42

71 Good, *The Steamer Parish*, p. 342

72 Good, *The Steamer Parish*, pp. 337–40; Worboys, 'The Colonial World'

73 MNA 47/LIM/1/1/35, Moffatt to Laws, 6 December 1918

74 Good, *The Steamer Parish*, p. 337, p. 341

75 For Malawi, see Hokkanen, *Medicine and the Scottish Missionaries*, p. 497. For collaboration within the wider Empire, see Ryan Johnson and Amna Khalid (eds.), *Public Health in the British Empire: Intermediaries, Subordinates, and the Practice of Public Health*, New York and London, Routledge, 2012

76 MNA 47/LIM/1/1/25a, Letterbook of Laws, 1925–1927, Laws to Superintendent of Census, 31 January 1925

77 Hokkanen, *Medicine and Scottish Missionaries*, pp. 497–8

78 Good, *The Steamer Parish*; Hokkanen, *Medicine and Scottish Missionaries*; Rennick, 'Church and Medicine'

79 Hokkanen, *Medicine and Scottish Missionaries*, pp. 414–18; King and King, *The Story of Medicine*, pp. 132–6

80 Nyasaland Protectorate, *Annual Medical Report for 1919*, Zomba, 1920

81 Nyasaland Protectorate, *Annual Medical Report for 1923*, Zomba, 1924

82 Nyasaland Protectorate, *Annual Medical Report for 1928*, Zomba, 1929, pp. 6, 23

83 King and King, *The Story of Medicine*, p. 136

84 MNA 47/LIM/1/19, Overtoun Institution Letterbook 1919–1921, letter 597, Laws to Innes, 28 April 1920. For a broader picture, see Johnson and Khalid (eds.), *Public Health in the British Empire*

85 TNA CO/626/8, Nyasaland Executive Council Minutes, 1926–1930, Minutes of the Executive Council, 19 August 1927

86 TNA CO/626/19, Nyasaland Protectorate Administration Reports, 1939, Annual Medical Report for 1939. Although Nyirenda and four others passed the Senior Hospital Assistant examination, only one (Dan Ngurube) was promoted in 1939

87 TNA CO/626/19, Nyasaland Protectorate Administration Reports, 1939, Annual Medical Report for 1939

88 Hokkanen, *Medicine and Scottish Missionaries*, pp. 415, 417; Nyasaland Protectorate, *Annual Medical Report for 1924*, Zomba, 1925, p. 17; Nyasaland Protectorate, *Annual Medical Report for 1930*, Zomba, 1931; King and King, *The Story of Medicine*, p. 133

89 Hokkanen, *Medicine and Scottish Missionaries*, pp. 414–18

90 Hokkanen, *Medicine and Scottish Missionaries*, pp. 420–1

91 NLS MS/7888, letter 98, Niven to Laws, 17 June 1925; MNA 47/LIM/1/1/25a, Letterbook of Laws 1925–1927, letter 45, Laws to Niven, no date

92 MNA 47/LIM/1/1/24, Letterbook of Laws, 1924–1925, letter 46, Laws to Chisholm, 4 November 1924

93 TNA CO/525/178/1, Minute of E.S. Boyd, 14 August 1939
94 TNA CO/626/19, Nyasaland Protectorate Administration Reports, 1939, Annual Report of the Social and Economic Progress of the People of Nyasaland for the Year 1939, p. 6
95 TNA CO/525/184/14, De Boer to Chief Secretary, 31 July 1940; Note of a talk with the Rev. H.M. Grace, 21 October 1940
96 TNA CO/525/177/17, Hall to the Under Secretary of State, Colonial Office, 15 August 1939
97 TNA CO/525/178/1, Minute of E.S. Boyd, 14 August 1939
98 MNA 47/LIM/1/1/14, Laws to Acting Chief Secretary, 2 August 1917; Hokkanen, *Medicine and Scottish Missionaries*, pp. 500–2
99 McCracken, *Politics and Christianity*, pp. 269–70; Hokkanen, *Medicine and Scottish Missionaries*, p. 502
100 TNA CO/525/184/14, Grace to the Under Secretary of State, Colonial Office, 16 September 1940
101 TNA CO/525/184/14, Grace to Sir Wilson Jameson, 22 October 1940
102 TNA CO/525/184/14, Note of a talk with the Rev. H.M. Grace, 21 October 1940
103 TNA CO/525/184/14, Jameson to De Boer, 22 October 1940
104 TNA CO/525/184/14, De Boer to Chief Secretary, 31 July 1940
105 TNA CO/525/184/14, Jameson to De Boer, 22 October 1940

CHAPTER FOUR

The maintenance of hegemony: the short history of Indian doctors in the Colonial Medical Service, British East Africa

Anna Greenwood and Harshad Topiwala

It is known that an increasing number of Indian doctors came to reside in the East African Protectorate (Kenya after 1920), following its formal colonisation by the British in 1895. What is less known, however, is that although some of these medical immigrants established themselves as private practitioners, the majority of them – at least in the period before 1923 – joined the Colonial Medical Service. Although these Indian practitioners were not appointed to the same rank as the European Medical Officers (MOs), they nevertheless were medically qualified individuals who had undergone training in Western medicine in India, usually for a minimum of three to five years, depending upon when and where the diploma or certificate was obtained.[1] Despite being awarded the less-prestigious rank of Assistant Surgeon, Sub-Assistant Surgeon (SAS) or Hospital Assistant within the Colonial Medical Service, and being paid lower salaries than MOs, these Indians to all intents and purposes fulfilled clinical roles and responsibilities similar to those of their European counterparts. Indeed, ample evidence exists that, before 1923, Indian practitioners were regarded as an invaluable constituent part of the medical infrastructure in the East African Protectorate. At their peak in 1920, there were almost twice as many Indian doctors as European MOs in the Government Medical Department. Furthermore, these men often took sole responsibility for regional hospitals, conducted large-scale disease surveys and serviced, without supervision, large and remote areas.[2]

This situation changed between 1922 and 1923, when the Indian contingent of the Colonial Medical Service was dramatically reduced by over a half in one year and the recruitment of Indian doctors abruptly stopped.[3] Suddenly, and largely without any detailed official explanation, Indians were dropped from the medical department staff lists and their work was no longer mentioned in colonial documentation. After more than two decades of successfully relying on Indian personnel, colonial officials silently, yet forcibly, wrote Indians out of the medical administration, and subsequently also out of later medical histories of this colonial possession.[4] Even the few Indian individuals that tenaciously remained in service in some of the outlying areas were no longer mentioned in the *Annual Medical Reports* or counted in departmental statistics.

Yet, as this chapter will show, the discreet turnabout in policy, although rarely mentioned in any official capacity at the time, can be quite easily explained retrospectively, most notably through tracing the several officially enshrined recommendations made against Indians in Kenya in the years immediately preceding 1923. Reports such as the 1919 Economic Commission Report, the 1922 Economic and Finance Committee Report (known as the Bowring Report) and the well-known 1923 Devonshire White Paper[5] all clearly set the scene for a newly hardened exclusionist attitude towards the participation of Indian immigrants in East African affairs. It was therefore quite in keeping with the mood of the time that official medical statements echoing these sentiments also appeared around this period. As we will discuss, the 1915 Simpson Report and the 1921 Public Health Ordinance provide two clear examples of this tendency.[6] Both documents explicitly condoned the implementation of segregative measures, justified on the grounds of the apparent link between Indians and poor hygiene. This was a new anti-Indian climate, fuelled partially by contemporaneous developments in other African territories (particularly South Africa), in which Indian workers and traders were increasingly portrayed as dirty and pathological bodies, while Indian doctors, precisely because they held some social status, were evidently felt to be challenging to white settler ideals of how the elite and responsible echelons of Kenyan society should be constituted.

Telling the little-known story about the way Indians were squeezed out of government positions offers valuable insights that can burst the historical myth of a Colonial Service staffed by the 'thin white line' famously described by Anthony Kirk-Greene in 1980.[7] Although, to be sure, the British colonial state in Africa principally consisted in its middle and higher echelons of white, elite personnel, in fact state representatives in roles of responsibility were sometimes of other nationalities and ethnicities. In short, non-whites were not limited to lower departmental staffing roles in the early history of the colonial medical department. Caught in the middle between the white elites and the (mostly) black subordinates, these Indian doctors became entirely overlooked in the medical history of Kenya. Even more recent moves to restore the often forgotten voices of the colonial nurses, subordinates and intermediaries to their rightful places within colonial history omit to mention this relatively large 'middle' cohort of qualified practitioners.[8]

Further, the short history of employing Indians within the colonial medical department shows that ideas of what was deemed appropriate in terms of representing the state locally were changeable. What was considered in one decade to be fitting to the times was evidently thought not to be appropriate in another. As such, this contribution to the history of Indians in the East African Colonial Medical Service highlights the way that colonial staffing policies were shaped by factors that went *beyond* the organisational effectiveness or the practical expediencies of the state (Indian doctors were cheap, Indian doctors had an acceptable level of training). Rather, the decision to squeeze Indians out of government employment was tied to changing social and political pressures that influenced ideas about the way the colonial project should be conducted. As ideas of trusteeship advanced from the 1920s, it became increasingly appropriate to Africanise the Colonial Medical Service, in terms of training and employing more African dressers; but at the same time (and with no apparent sense of contradiction) as the Service became more inclusive towards Africans, it became less inclusive towards Indians. This implies that, despite British rhetoric, something more complicated than progressive racial inclusion was going on. In key ways, Indians working in roles similar to those of Europeans in Africa posed a threat to British ideas of colonial hegemony.

Indians, migration and medicine

The migration of Indians to East Africa has been the subject of much scholarly attention, although no work has concentrated upon medical migration per se.[9] Between 1900 and 1948, more than 150,000 Indians settled in the East African colonies, although this trend for Indians to seek opportunities in the area was far from new.[10] Evidence from as early as AD 120 suggests the movement of people and trade between the Indian subcontinent and the African East Coast, and by the thirteenth century trading excursions by both Indians and Arabs to the African coast were commonplace, with dhows regularly moving between the shores of India, the Persian Gulf and East Africa using the seasonal winds.[11] Much of the early trade centred upon the island of Zanzibar, which for several centuries was the regional hub of trade, particularly in slaves, ivory and spices. Although much of the commerce was in the hands of the wealthy Omani elite, Indians were vital cogs in the commercial successes of the region and Indian models of business organisation came to be highly esteemed by both the Portuguese colonisers of Zanzibar in the sixteenth and seventeenth centuries and the Omani rulers who subsequently came to power in 1698.[12] Through several centuries of trading contact, Indians had come to know the geography of the region well and were key players in both local and international commerce. As such, they became relied upon as organisers of potentially risky caravan expeditions into the interior, and also as financiers in trading initiatives to both India and the Americas.[13]

By the time the British arrived in East Africa in 1888 with the Imperial British East Africa Company (IBEAC), a sizeable Indian community already resided along the coast and its adjacent islands. The presence of this resident community, combined with the colonial power that Britain already wielded in the Indian subcontinent, meant that it was no surprise that Britain looked to Indians as key personnel to aid in the establishment and consolidation of power in its new Protectorate.[14] From the mid-1890s Indian army regiments were brought in to secure military control, and between 1898 and 1902 approximately 31,000 indentured labourers from India were employed to expedite the first major colonial construction project in the region, the Uganda Railway – stretching from the coastal city of Mombasa to the edges of inland Lake Victoria.[15]

At the formation of the IBEAC the directors had positioned themselves on this issue:

> The question of immigration from India appears to the Directors to be of great importance, with a view to colonisation by trained agriculturalists of the unoccupied districts of the Company's territory, more notably at Witu, in the country between the Tana and Juba Rivers and in the Sabaki Valley where the climate, soil and general conditions are particularly favourable to their settlement. The entire trade of East Africa has long been carried on by wealthy resident British Indian merchants, themselves large plantation owners, who would greatly welcome and encourage their countrymen to settle in Africa. The Directors have under consideration the expediency of initiating the movement by offering grants of unoccupied lands to approved families. With such support and encouragement Africa may in future become to the natives of India what America and the British colonies have proved to the mother country and Europe.[16]

Others shared these views. During the early years of the Protectorate many respected colonial experts, including Sir Bartle Frere, John Ainsworth and Harry Johnston, the Special Commissioner for Uganda, also put forward compelling reasons for promoting Indian settlement in East Africa.[17]

It is in the light of this context of enthusiasm that the early employment of Indians in the colonial medical department can be understood. The early Indian doctors, since 1897, hailed from a mix of Indian communities, although Christians, including Goans, (if available), were preferred by the British administration for their adoption of European habits.[18] Concurrently, Indian doctors were also employed in other capacities supportive to British colonialism: they were imported to serve the health of the Indian regiments billeted in East Africa, and also to provide basic medical services to the thousands of indentured Indian labourers working on the Uganda Railway.[19]

Western medical education in India

One of the reasons why Indian doctors were employed was because they provided relatively cheap labour, but nevertheless medical labour that had been trained in standards comparable (although never deemed equal) to those on offer in medical schools in the West. A comprehensive history of the development of Western medical education in India remains to be written, but some regional accounts of medical professionalisation provide useful insights, showing clearly that Western medical education became well established in India by the mid-nineteenth century.[20] Calcutta Medical College opened its doors in February 1835 as the first institution explicitly designed to train young Indian boys, irrespective of caste, in the principles of Western medicine in English. By 1846 qualifications earned from this college were formally recognised by the London Royal College of Surgeons, and by 1857, the year in which the institution was confirmed as having full university status, Licentiate in Medicine and Surgery (LMS), Bachelor in Medicine (MB) and Doctor of Medicine (MD) were all offered, in line with the medical degrees available in the UK.[21]

The Western medical education established at Calcutta was soon copied elsewhere. Madras Medical College admitted its first students in 1842; Grant Medical College in Bombay (a key provider of doctors for Kenya) in 1845; and Lahore Medical School (also called King Edward Medical School) was established in 1860.[22]

One confusing issue was that, upon qualification from a medical school in India, there was little systematisation in terms of how these newly qualified practitioners were titled.[23] Deeply rooted ideas of racial superiority in the Colonial Service meant that Indian colleagues, even if in possession of LMS or MD degrees, were seldom allowed the job title of Medical Officer, which was reserved mainly for Europeans. Instead, Indian medical graduates were variously called Assistant Surgeons, SASs and even sometimes Hospital Assistants once they took up posts with the British government services. Although the higher-ranked Assistant Surgeons are usually relatively easy to identify, before the Medical Registration Ordinance of 1910, SASs were sometimes also referred to as Hospital Assistants. This variety of job titles means that, especially in the first decade of the colonial medical department in East Africa, it is difficult to tell from the job title whether the individual mentioned was a doctor with a General Medical Council recognised medical degree or a medical subordinate with a less prestigious diploma or a certificate.[24] The disparities in nomenclature are revealing both of the lower status that Britain attributed to Indian medical qualifications and also of deeply embedded racial beliefs that ultimately saw the true leaders of the British Empire as white.

Indians in the Colonial Medical Service before 1923

In East Africa, Indian Assistant Surgeons and SASs were present in the medical department as an obvious force soon after its inception. Indians were part of the medical provision offered by the Uganda Railways and then, later, part of the colonial medical department, which was founded in 1895. Although official records from this period are scant, four Indian medical staff are named in early archive material before 1900: Edward Oorloff, who had joined the medical department in 1897; E.W. Rodrigo and G.P. Vinod, who had served since 1898; and Maula Buksh who joined the department in 1899.[25] It was apparent from very early on that, even if the healthcare focus was primarily on the needs of the European community, few European doctors were available and the department relied on supplementary staffing.[26] Correspondence between Kenya, London and India confirms a heavy dependence on Indian staff for the provision of medical services, with numerous examples in the records of calls to secure more Indian doctors.[27] In 1921, even John Langton Gilks, the Principal Medical Officer (PMO) who was to actively squeeze Indians out of Colonial Medical Service employment, had drawn attention to the problem of the Indian medical staff being 'inconveniently low'.[28]

As might be expected, conditions of employment for the assistant surgeons and SASs were less favourable than those offered to European MOs. Although both groups had their passage to East Africa paid, the salaries offered were far from equivalent and the allowances were very different. While European MOs were paid £400 *per annum* (in 1939 this changed to £600 *per annum*), the salary of an Assistant Surgeon was approximately £200 and that of an SAS (or Hospital Assistant) was under £70.[29] Furthermore, unlike the European doctors, who were provided with government housing, subordinate Indian staff had neither an accommodation allowance nor guaranteed government housing, no gratuity for long service, no passages paid for spouses and family and no formal provision was made for their pension, unless they first passed a three-year probationary period.[30]

For almost three decades, Indian Assistant Surgeons and SASs were the vital cogs in the machinery of the Government Medical Department. In fact, in the years before 1923, all the available evidence indicates that Indian doctors were present in equal or greater numbers than their European counterparts. At their high point in 1919, almost twice as many Indian practitioners (seventy-three) worked for the East African Colonial Medical Service as did Europeans (forty-three) – a fact that makes their omission from the subsequent histories of medicine in East Africa all the more remarkable. Although a rhetoric of economic saving was cited as justification for the drastic cull of Indian personnel in 1922, it is thought-provoking that European staffing numbers, after a small reduction in 1923, nevertheless steadily grew from 1925 to almost double in the 1930s, despite the fact that European MO salaries were much higher than those offered to Assistant Surgeons or SASs.[31]

Colonial Medical Service doctors[32]

The lack of source material makes it difficult to gain a full picture of the typical experiences of Indian doctors.[33] Similar to European doctors, most Indian doctors posted outside of the main townships conducted very independent professional lives, able to make their own decisions, and often responsible at a comparatively early stage of their careers for thousands of patients.[34] District medical reports for 1915–23 from Meru, 1914–22 in Malindi and 1921 in Kabarnet give an indication of the high levels of responsibility many Indian subordinate doctors had.[35] Many of the Indian subordinate doctors were in sole charge of hospitals and managed sizable staff. For instance, an Indian Assistant Surgeon was responsible for the hospital at Fort Hall during 1919 and an SAS was in charge of the Machakos hospital in the Ukamba reserve for several years before 1922.[36] Although theoretically Indian subordinates were always under the supervision of the local MO, in reality those in remote locations were only infrequently visited, in some instances only once a year.[37] Furthermore, evidence can be found that some of the Indian members of the Colonial Medical Service were actively engaged in medical research. Between 1922 and 1940 fifteen different Indian medical department colleagues contributed to the *Kenya Medical Journal* (after 1932, *East African Medical Journal*), reporting on topics as varied as pellagra, pneumonia, surgical methods and memory loss. Some individuals undertook large surveys of their local African communities and were committed to the improvement of standards of care and the expansion of knowledge about African diseases and their mitigating factors. For example the 1913 *Annual Medical Report* describes in significant detail the anti-plague campaigns of three Indian doctors,

A.N. Nyss, K.H. Bhatt and Murari Lal.[38] Another article, from 1927, by Assistant Surgeon T.D. Nair, described his extensive yaws eradication campaign along the Tana River.[39] A medical report authored by Minoo Dastur reveals in vivid detail his substantial initiatives to improve public health provision in the Baringo district of Kenya.[40]

Before the 1920s it is not difficult to find positive comments concerning the use of Indian subordinate doctors. Individuals working in East Africa, India and the UK regularly praised the quality of Indian staff. E.B. Horne, who was the District Officer in Meru, for example, was immensely impressed by the performance of Abdulla Khan, who commenced work in Meru in 1915, describing his 'relations with the natives' as 'excellent'. Horne further commented that because of Khan's professional efforts and good personal relations there had been a substantive increase in patient consultations under his tenure.[41] Similarly, the author of a report issued in 1921 concerning the remote Kabarnet station, which was considered to have 'deplorable' facilities and to be 'notoriously unhealthy', made strikingly appreciative comments about the improvements that occurred in the health of the region under the Indian doctor's charge.[42] Six months after Gokul Chand's appointment to the station, the District Commissioner was happy to report that 'his work has been eminently satisfactory, the sanitation of the station is looked after by him with great care'.[43]

In his published reminiscences of 1928 in the *Kenya and East African Medical Journal*, former PMO Arthur Milne also extolled the contribution of Indian doctors, along with those of Goan clerks, in glowing terms, describing them as 'the two main-springs which have kept the wheels of the department turning'.[44] He singled out a number of individuals for their gallantry and dedication to the establishment of colonial medicine in the region, describing Assistant Surgeon de Cruz as one of the 'never to be forgotten comrades who laid down their lives in building up of these colonies'.[45] Other European MOs provided similar positive testaments of the Indian medical staff. Robert Hennessey made particular note of the vital role of the Indian doctors in the running of the hospitals and their importance in undertaking much of the routine surgery.[46] Another senior European MO, Peter Clearkin, who worked for some time at Kisumu Hospital, described some of the Assistant Surgeons whom he worked with as 'very good indeed', making specific reference to the outstanding efforts of one individual, Kartar Singh.[47]

The demise of Indian Colonial Medical Service careers

Although by the early 1920s it seemed that Indians were an integral part of the colonial medical administration, the glowing endorsements of their service came to an end in 1922. The reason for this abrupt turnabout in attitudes was never articulated beyond generalised statements about the need to enforce economies within the department, some comments about the new preference to Africanise the Colonial Medical Service, and a few references to the alleged lack of suitability of Indians to perform medical duties for Africans.

Although a number of short-term factors can be identified as inducing this policy shift, in many important ways the groundwork for this sea-change in attitudes had been gradually established since the beginning of the twentieth century. Despite the apparent enthusiasm for the employment of Indian doctors before 1922, nearly every positive remark about them was nevertheless made in a climate that concurrently also assumed that Indians were neither as able nor as desirable as European doctors. Kenya, with its politically powerful white settler community, was particularly a place where Indians were routinely discriminated against. The prominent roles some Indians played in business and commerce in the region made settlers not only suspicious of the possibility of Indian encroaching political power but also desirous to limit it at every available opportunity. Frequent portrayals of Indians in the settler-led local press made allusion to their thrift and business acumen, characteristics which were portrayed not as qualities to be praised but as traits of which other members of the colonial community should be suspicious.[48] Running alongside this discourse, with apparently no sense of contradiction, was another prominent stereotype propagated by the British, namely that Indians, particularly those of poor socio-economic standing, were a public health risk and were therefore actually a threat to the prosperity of the colony. Sentiments such as 'whenever one finds the Indian in Africa, he appears so dirty' were commonplace and profoundly affected the way Indians were regarded not only as patients, but also as doctors.[49] Prominent European doctors, such as Roland Burkitt, supported this view, even publicly lecturing on the allegedly deplorable habits of Indians and making no attempt to disguise their hostility towards the community.[50]

In addition to this climate of gradually increasing racial animosity to the East African Indian community since 1900, several tangible points can be identified as marking significant stepping-stones on the path to outright hostility. One of the most dramatic shifts in attitude can be pinpointed to the change in Commissionership (Governorship after 1906) in 1900 from Sir Arthur Hardinge to Sir Charles Eliot. This marked the concerted beginnings of the 'White Highlands Policy', which favoured the white settlement of the area located to the north of Nairobi and the west of Mount Kenya, which was thought to have the most fertile land and the most agreeable climate.

[72]

During his time as Commissioner of the East Africa Protectorate (1895–1900) Hardinge had established a model of colonial administration that drew heavily on Indian personnel, not only as indentured labourers but also as he sought staff in positions of responsibility, such as at the head of the Works and Transport departments.[51] While Hardinge was agreed that the Highlands would be the best place for white settlement, he nevertheless accepted Indian landownership as part of the cultural landscape of the East Africa Protectorate.[52] When Eliot succeeded to the headship of the Protectorate it was quite clear that his sympathies were elsewhere. His candid statement of 1905 could not have been further away from the integrationist ideas of his predecessor: 'I think it is a mere hypocrisy not to admit that white interests must be paramount, and the main object of our policy and legislation should be to found a white colony.'[53]

Immediately upon his investiture Eliot drove a private bargain with the leader of the 'white frontiersmen' of Kenya, Lord Delamere, and invited Europeans including, White South Africans, to migrate.[54] Eliot was to be only the first of a series of governors to fall 'willingly into settler clutches'.[55] Many of his successors, including Sir Edouard Girouard (1909–12), Sir Henry Belfield (1912–17), Sir Charles Bowring (1917–19) and Sir Edward Northey (1919–22), displayed sympathy for the settler position and, increasingly, an accompanying disregard for the Indian community of East Africa.[56]

Towards the end of the First World War the issue of whether Indians should be awarded land grants in East Africa in formal recognition of their contribution to the war effort was seriously discussed. The subject was considered so important that it became the subject of parliamentary debate in London, but nevertheless the motion eventually suffered a crushing defeat, with settler opposition to the proposal playing no small part in its decisive demise.[57] During the next four years, undoubtedly in the light of fears raised through the serious discussions about possible land grants for Indians, a number of blatantly anti-Indian reports were produced concerning Kenya colony.

The first such document came in the form of the findings of the Economic Commission of 1919. This Commission had been set up by Governor Belfield with the specific aim to inquire and report on a sustainable future for the colony. The conclusions of the final report of this commission were unambiguous:

Physically, the Indian is not a wholesome influence because of his incurable repugnance to sanitation and hygiene....The moral depravity of the Indian is equally damaging to the African, who in his natural state is at least innocent of the worst vices of the East. The Indian is the inciter to crime as well as vice, ...The presence of the Indian in this country is quite obviously inimical to the moral and physical welfare and the economic advancement of the native.[58]

The final recommendations of the report explicitly stated that senior posts in government, railway, municipalities and European firms should be reserved exclusively for Europeans. Among its recommendations were a complete halt to Indian immigration and a call that all government departments 'should, as quickly as possible replace Indian employees by Europeans in the higher grades and Africans in the lower'.[59] Indians were described as displaying an aversion to sanitation and hygiene and as having disproportionately large numbers of their community associated with crime and vice.[60] With the findings of the 1919 Economic Commission, anti-Indian sentiment within East Africa palpably strengthened. Calls started to be made by both settlers and members of colonial government demanding the complete cessation of Indian immigration and the transfer of Indian-held jobs in government to Europeans and Africans, in line with the Commission's recommendations.[61]

This new, unambiguously exclusionist line of argumentation was further reiterated with the findings of the 1922 Economic and Finance Committee (Bowring Committee). This committee, which had been set up along the lines of the Geddes Committee in the UK to evaluate the need to reduce public expenditure and introduce protective tariffs in the colony, proposed in its conclusions a 20 per cent reduction in the number of all Asiatic civil servants working for the British government in East Africa.[62] With seemingly no sense of contradiction, this projected staff reduction was justified on the grounds of ameliorating the deteriorating financial situation of the colony. Indian leaders were quick to point out the illogicality of removing Indian staff as 'the salaries of some of the Asiatic staff are at present less than a quarter of the minimum salaries drawn by European staff' who were being retained, but this reasoning appeared to carry no weight in a colonial administration determined, under settler pressure, to reduce the influence of the Indian community.[63] The budget cuts recommended in the Bowring Committee Report inflicted the biggest hardships on Indians, who were deemed to be too expensive and not suitable to work in the colonial administration. It was stated that it would be more economical to replace Indians gradually with cheaper African labour and, furthermore, that only Europeans could act as trustees for the Africans, who were not yet considered to be in a position to represent their own interests. Indians were regarded as being fundamentally unsuitable for colonial service, as they could not provide the necessary moral and social guidance to the majority African community.

Finally, the most decisive watershed was to occur in the following year, in the form of the 1923 Devonshire White Paper.[64] The debates leading up to, and during, the passing of the Devonshire Declaration have been the subject of extensive scholarship and it is necessary here just to summarise its main conclusions.[65]

The Devonshire Declaration signified the formal pronouncement of the British government's intentions for Kenya colony. Native rights were to be paramount in the long term and, in order to prepare the indigenous population for self-rule, European interim trusteeship was to be the short-term focus. In this framework there was little space for Indian rights (similar to those enjoyed by Europeans). Indians were not seen as the natural inhabitants of Kenya, neither through inheritance nor conquest, and their rights to political representation were severely curbed. There would be no common franchise. Indians were to be allowed five elected seats in the Legislative Council, compared to eleven for Europeans. Additionally, Devonshire confirmed that the Highlands would be reserved for Europeans and the option of a future ban on Indian immigration was maintained.

The anti-Indian sentiments which manifested themselves in the recommendations of the Economic Commission, the Bowring Committee and the Devonshire Declaration also permeated colonial medical policy in areas of public health: the Simpson Report of 1915 and the Public Health Ordinance of 1921. The Simpson Report came about as a direct result of the frequent complaints about the sanitary condition of Nairobi, particularly stimulated by objections to the insanitary state of the Indian bazaar. In response to these issues, Governor Henry Belfield in 1912 sought the help of a sanitation expert to provide a professional assessment of the situation. Professor W.J. Simpson, a member of the Advisory Committee on Tropical Medicine, was the natural choice for the job. By the time of his appointment he had already been on missions to investigate sanitary conditions in Gold Coast, Sierra Leone and Nigeria on behalf of the British colonial government.[66] Simpson visited Kenya in 1914, travelling extensively throughout the country for six months. In compiling his assessment he drew upon many interviews, although notably few with non-Europeans.[67]

Simpson's final report of 1915, illustrated with town plans and photographs, was unambiguous in its support of racial segregation and became much cited as official justification for colonial health policies thereafter. He was unswerving in his recommendations:

Lack of control over buildings, streets and lanes, and over the general growth and development of towns and trade centres in East Africa and Uganda, combined with the intermingling, in the same quarters of town and trade centres of races with different customs and habits, accounts for many of the insanitary conditions in them and for the extension of disease from one race to another.... Also ... the diseases to which these different races are respectively liable are readily transferable to the European and vice versa, a result specially liable to occur when their dwellings are near each other.... [I]t is absolutely essential that in every town and trade centre the town planning should provide well defined and separate quarters or wards for Europeans, Asiatics and Africans ... and that there should be a neutral belt of open unoccupied country of at least 300 yards in width between European residences and those of the Asiatic and African.[68]

Although not accepted without controversy, the Simpson Report became used as the authoritative medical reference to defend East African Protectorate policies of racial segregation. It became the basis for the first comprehensive Public Health Ordinance of 1921, which was instructed as means to simplify navigation of the numerous health ordinances against specific diseases or procedures that had been accumulating in the Protectorate since its earliest days.[69] The story of the passage of this Ordinance is long and complicated, but ultimately the British government rejected clause 15, which advocated racial segregation along the lines recommended by Simpson in 1915.[70] Nevertheless, the debates over the inclusion of this clause and the evident enthusiasm for segregation among members of the settler community show how urgent the need to limit Indian rights was perceived to be by some sectors of the colonial community. It was no surprise that racial segregation of township areas in Kenya did not end with the removal of clause 15. Europeans found other ways of maintaining *de facto* segregation and the administration did little to intervene and ensure compliance. Instead, subtle ways were found to conform to most resident Europeans' preferences to live in a segregated society, for example by turning down planning applications by non-Europeans and refusing to sell land to Indians. Officials in Whitehall were aware that the law was being circumvented, but were content to turn a blind eye. A handwritten comment on an internal Colonial Office memorandum is revealing: tacit support of these continued practices of segregation was provided as long as a way could be found 'of avoiding official correspondence' on the subject.[71]

The final piece in the jigsaw in understanding the dramatic retrenchment of more than half of all Indian staff from the Colonial Medical Service lies in the actions of the PMO at that time – John Langton Gilks. Although, to be sure, Gilks was influenced by the broader social and political environment around him, it was his eventual support for the scheme which directly lay behind the fact that many Indians lost their jobs in 1922. Gilks was extremely cautious of recording in any detail the impetuses behind his policy decisions, and his motives can only be guessed at through relatively limited evidence. Enough evidence exists, however, to verify that he became a close ally of the Kenyan settler community and that his views about Indians for the most part accorded with the dominant settler mood of negativity towards them.[72] Despite initial wavering on Gilks's part, Legislative and Executive Council minutes record his ultimate acquiescence to the segregation of Indians in townships and the reduction of non-European salaries and his support for communal voting, which all Indians vehemently opposed.[73] He additionally refused to back a proposal to grant licensed Indian doctors a permanent right to practise medicine provided that they had completed three years' satisfactory medical service in the colony. Gilks openly criticised the quality of medical degrees from India, stating that 'certain degrees [of India] were not recognised. All sub assistants were not good doctors and some were not fit to practise without supervision.'[74] In his short, characteristically dry, memoirs of his time in Kenya, Gilks referred to the staffing reductions only as a means of achieving the economic savings recommended by the Bowring Committee. The second pretext he put forward for the action in 1922 was that, under the new priorities of trusteeship, Indians were unsuited to colonial medical work because the 'inclinations of these Indian SASs were not towards the care of Africans' and their withdrawal from the outstations 'would not appear to have been followed by serious results'.[75]

This was a theme that was echoed in other quarters. The local branch of the British Medical Association (BMA) was much less reticent in vocalising its support for the policy to cull Indians from the Colonial Medical Service.[76] In a memorandum to the London-based Dominions Committee the Kenya branch of the BMA declared:

A specific question having been asked by the Commission as to the efficiency of Indian sub-assistant surgeons, the Branch wishes to express the opinion that though they may fulfil a useful function when working under the supervision of medical officers, yet, owing to their attitude towards the African they are as a rule unsatisfactory for independent medical work amongst natives. At the time of retrenchment the establishment of sub assistant surgeons was greatly reduced. This was a step in the right direction and the Branch considers that the eventual replacement of Asiatics is desirable. The replacement of an Asiatic sub-assistant surgeon in charge of an outstation by a medical officer entails additional expense yet the increase in value of the public health service rendered is out of all proportion to the increase in cost.[77]

Furthermore, the new, pressing priority was to Africanise colonial medicine, so it is no coincidence that the scheme to employ Africans in larger numbers was promoted in earnest in 1924, less than two years after Indian staffing was cut.[78] Indeed, the increase in numbers of African dressers within the colonial medical department was dramatic: numbers rose from a handful in 1920 to 648 fifteen years later.[79] By 1932 more than 1,000 Africans were said to be working for the colonial medical department, over half of them categorised as dressers.[80]

A reduced number of Indian Assistant Surgeons and SASs continued to operate in rural East African locations, despite the official cull. In 1937, an annual report indicated that a third of the hospitals in the African reserves were still under the charge of an Indian doctor, though they were barely mentioned in government reports.[81] A few tenacious Indian doctors, even if they were largely ignored and severely depleted in numbers, formed a constituent part of the colonial department. It is difficult to gauge their relative contribution, but estimates collated for 1937 suggest that twenty-six continued to operate in the country, with more than half in outlying regions.

Conclusion

Although accounts left by Indian members of the medical service are few and evidence has had to be pulled together from disparate sources, it is still possible to build up a picture of the short history of Indian doctors in the Colonial Medical Service.[82] Indian doctors, although employed on less favourable contractual terms – and typically posted to the less popular, remote stations – nevertheless were an extremely valuable part of the health service infrastructure, easily outnumbering European doctors during the first twenty-five years of the colonial medical department.

The disappearance of Indian doctors from the record after 1923 in large part explains their disappearance from colonial medical history. Indeed, reading the currently available literature, one might be forgiven for assuming that the East African Colonial Medical Service was entirely staffed by white, European doctors.[83] It is hoped that the new insights offered by this study will extend understandings not only through providing more empirical data about how the Colonial Service was staffed, but also in terms of helping historians to reflect on the processes of recording history; ones that sometimes bury important aspects for generations. The policy of dropping Indians from the Colonial Medical Service was rarely directly spoken about at the time, which meant that subsequently their history also became overlooked. This story provides a cautionary tale: in the struggle to escape the positivist, triumphalist white histories of the early post-colonial era more recent historical attention has refocused our interests on the history of black participation in Empire.[84] Understandably, but inevitably too simplistically, the history of the black African doctors was assumed to be the only crucial missing part of the story.[85] In fact, the way Empire was staffed in East Africa was more nuanced. Although Indians were themselves divided as a group and should by no means be seen as homogeneous in opinion and stance towards the British government (or even towards members of their own community), omitting their contribution to the East African Colonial Medical Service fails to acknowledge some of the diversity of the British Empire and some of the subtleties within the colonial politics of race.

The contextual analysis offered in this chapter shows that of the events around 1923 are (retrospectively at least) explicable, if they were surreptitiously conducted. The abrupt change in official attitudes towards Indians in the Colonial Medical Service shows that broader social and political dynamics were at play in decisions about their large-scale retrenchment. While it became acceptable – perhaps precisely because it was relatively non-threatening – to provide training for indigenous Africans as dressers and Hospital Assistants, the idea of working side by side with similarly qualified Indian individuals had less political appeal. This prospect became progressively more problematic after the First World War, when the potentially destabilising effects of increased Indian social and political influence were hotly debated issues within East Africa and Indians became increasingly cast in official reports (such as the 1919 Economic Commission Report, the 1922 Bowring Report and the 1923 Devonshire White Paper) as a potentially large public nuisance whose ambitions were to be curtailed before they got out of hand. The British government could not risk alienating the powerful white settler community, so, while limiting the worst excesses of their demands, it also tacitly understood the importance of keeping policies at a level in accordance, at least nominally, with settler desires. In this way, looking beyond the immediate boundaries of medical priorities or organisational efficiency, the decision to drastically reduce Indian members of the Colonial Medical Service can be better understood. Despite almost three decades of good service, educated Indian doctors were ultimately feared as a threat to British dominance in Kenya.[86]

Notes

1   British Library (BL) IOR/L/MIL/7/5334 Collection 116/62 Minutes of the Indian Legislative Assembly, 2 May 1924, pp. 1905, 1966; The National Archives, UK (TNA) CO/535/3 Correspondence, Dr Donaldson, Senior Medical Officer to Governor of Somaliland, 6 May–24 July 1933

2   'Assistant Surgeon Nyss in Charge of Plague Camps', *Annual Medical Department Report, East African Protectorate (AMR)*, 1914, p. 89. See also *AMR*, 1913, p. 78

[79]

3   The cull is fleetingly mentioned in: John Langton Gilks, 'The Medical Department and the Health Organization of Kenya, 1909–1933', *The East African Medical Journal*, 9, 1932–33, pp. 340–54, at p. 350. Earlier, the 1922 *AMR* detailed the reductions to make economies and listed the closure of eleven out stations in the charge of Sub-Assistant Surgeons.

4   Ann Beck, *A History of the British Medical Administration of East Africa, 1900–1950*, Cambridge, MA, Harvard University Press, 1970; Megan Vaughan, *Curing Their Ills: Colonial Power and African Illness*, Cambridge, Polity Press, 1991; John Iliffe, *East African Doctors: a History of the Modern Profession*, Cambridge, Cambridge University Press, 1998; Anna Crozier, *Practising Colonial Medicine: the Colonial Medical Service in East Africa*, London, I.B. Tauris, 2007

5   BL IOR/L/PJ/6/1718 *Economic Commission Report*, Nairobi, Swift Press, 1919; BL IOR/L/E/7/1264 'Indians in Kenya', The Devonshire Declaration, White Paper, Cmd. 1922, July 1923. No copy of the Bowring Report has been located: second-hand reporting of its findings in other sources has been used throughout.

6   W.J. Simpson, *Report on the Sanitary Matters in the East Africa Protectorate, Uganda and Zanzibar*, London, Colonial Office, Africa No. 1025, February 1915; Kenya Colony, Public Health Ordinance, Nairobi, Kenya, Government Printers, 1921.

7   See Anthony M. Kirk-Greene, 'The Thin White Line: The Size of the British Colonial Service in Africa', *African Affairs*, 79, 1980, pp. 25–44

8   See chapters relating to Africa in Ryan Johnson and Amna Khalid (eds.), *Public Health in the British Empire: Intermediaries, Subordinates, and the Practice of Public Health*, New York and London, Routledge, 2012; Anne Digby, *Diversity and Division in Medicine: Healthcare in South Africa from the 1800s*, Oxford, Peter Lang, 2006

9   Uchhrangrai Keshavrai Oza, *The Rift in the Empire's Lute: Being a History of the Indian Struggle in Kenya from 1900 to 1930*, Nairobi, Advocate of India Press, 1930; Lawrence William Hollingsworth, *The Asians of East Africa*, London, Macmillan and Co. Ltd., 1960; George Delf, *Asians in East Africa*, Oxford, Oxford University Press, 1963; J.S. Mangat, *A History of the Asians in East Africa, c.1886–1945*, Oxford, Oxford University Press, 1969; Dharam P. Ghai and Yash P. Ghai (eds.), *Portrait of a Minority: Asians in East Africa*, Nairobi and London, Oxford University Press, 1970; Robert G. Gregory, *India and East Africa: A History of Race Relations within the British Empire, 1890–1939*, Oxford, Clarendon Press, 1971; Agehananda Bharati, *The Asians in East Africa: Jayhind and Uhuru*, Chicago, Nelson-Hall Co., 1972; Cynthia Salvadori, *We Came in Dhows*, 3 vols, Nairobi, Paperchase Kenya Ltd, 1996

10 C.J. Martin, 'A Demographic Study of an Immigrant Community: The Indian Population of British East Africa', *Population Studies*, 6, 3, 1953, pp. 233–47

11 Some of this early evidence before Vasco de Gama's voyage of 1497 is disputed and inconclusive. R. Coupland, *East Africa and its Invaders from the Earliest Times to the Death of Seyyid Said*, London, Oxford University Press, 1938, p. 16; Gregory, *India and East Africa*, pp. 9–15; M.N. Pearson, *Port Cities and Intruders: The Swahili Coast, India and Portugal in the Early Modern Era*, Baltimore, MD, Johns Hopkins University Press, 1998, p. 11

12 M. Reda Bhacker, *Trade and Empire in Muscat and Zanzibar: The Roots of British Domination*, London, Routledge, 1992, p. 12

13 Rhodes House Library, Oxford (RHL) MSS.Brit.Emp.s.22G5 IBEAC, Sir Francis de Winton, memorandum, 18 August 1890; see also quotation from Sir Bartle Frere in T.M. Metcalf, *Imperial Connections: India in the Indian Ocean Arena, 1860–1920*, Berkeley and London, University of California Press, 2007, p. 166

14 Mangat, *History of the Asians in East Africa*, p. 28

15 The precise figure quoted by Gregory is 31,983, *India and East Africa*, p. 52

16 RHL MSS.Brit.Emp.s.22G5 IBEAC, Report of the Court of Directors to the Annual Shareholders Meeting, 27 July 1891, p. 4; Gregory, *India and East Africa*, p. 49

17 Frere is cited in Mangat, *History of the Asians in East Africa*, p. 12; similarly, Ainsworth's comments on the positive role of Indians can be seen in his farewell speech reported in *East African Chronicle*, 14 August 1920, p. 14; See also Harry Johnson, Letter to the Editor, *The Times*, 22 August 1921, p. 4; BL IOR/L/PJ/6/807 shows that in 1907 Churchill also refused to rule out Indian settlement from the Highlands.

18 TNA CO/544/14, Kenya Executive Council Minutes, 1918, p. 363, where mention is made of bonus awards to Assistant Surgeons 'who looked and behaved as English gentlemen'; the essential role of Goan clerks together with Indian subordinate doctors in the administration of the Medical Department was also pointed out in Arthur Dawson Milne, 'The Rise of the Colonial Medical Service', *Kenya and East African Medical Journal*, 5, 1928–29, pp. 50–8, at p. 58

19 Because of the scant evidence available for this period, regrettably, not a great deal is known about the background, precise qualifications and activities of Indian medical men working for the British military in East Africa. Nevertheless, some positive comments about Indian medical contributions can be found, occasionally naming names. See, for example: BL IOR/L/MIL/7/2188 and BL IOR/L/MIL/7/2189, Despatch 2 March 1899 (outlining military awards to six named individuals, including the Indian MO in charge, Surgeon Lt H.M. Masani, and Hospital Assistants B. Kasinath, Maula Baksh, Rahim Baksh, Sheikh Ahmed and Niyamtullah); W. Lloyd-Jones, *K.A.R.: Being an Unofficial Account of the Origin and Activities of the King's African Rifles*, London, Arrowsmith, 1926, pp. 48, 64; W. Lloyd-Jones, *Havash Frontier Adventures in Kenya*, London, Arrowsmith, 1925, p. 290. A little more is available on Indian doctors working for the Uganda Railway. See BL IOR/MIL/7/2153 Indian Hospital Assistants accompanying the Railway Survey, 1891; BL IOR/MIL/7/2175 and BL IOR/MIL/7/2188 Recruitment of Medical Staff for Railways, 1895–6, 1897–9; BL IOR/MIL/7/14462 Rahmat Ali Petition, 24 May 1899

20 Poonam Bala, *Imperialism and Medicine in Bengal*, New Delhi, Sage Publications, 1991; V.R. Muraleedharan, 'Professionalising Medical Practice in Colonial South India', *Economic and Political Weekly*, 27, 4, 1992; pp. PE27–30, PE35–7; Mridula Ramanna, *Western Medicine and Public Health in Colonial Bombay, 1845–1895*, Delhi, Orient Longman, 2002; M. Gopal, D. Balasubramanian, P. Kanagarajah, A. Anirudhan and P. Murugan, 'Madras Medical College, 175 Years of Medical Heritage', *The National Medical Journal of India*, 23, 2, 2010, pp. 117–20

21 Calcutta Medical College, *The Centenary of the Medical College, Bengal, 1835–1934*, Calcutta, Calcutta Medical College, 1935; Bala, *Imperialism and Medicine in Bengal*; S.N. Sen, *Scientific and Technical Education in India 1781–1900*, New Delhi, Indian National Science Academy, 1991

22 Gopal et al. 'Madras Medical College'; Abdur Pashid, *History of the King Edward Medical College Lahore, 1860–1960*, Lahore, 1960

23 Another potentially confusing issue lies in trying to distinguish Indian Christians, Goans, Eurasians and Europeans by their names alone. It is theoretically possible, although unlikely, that some of the Assistant Surgeons listed *may* have been Europeans born in India.

24 'An Ordinance to make Provision for the Registration of Medical Practitioners and Dentists through the 1910 Medical Practitioners and Dentists Ordinance', *The Official Gazette*, 1 October 1910, p. 575

25 BL, microfilm, Government Publications Relating to Kenya, 1897–1963, East African Protectorate Blue Book, 1901/1902

26 H.A. Bödeker, 'Some Sidelights on Early Medical History in East Africa', *The East African Medical Journal*, 12, 1935–36, pp. 100–7, at p. 105

27 BL IOR/MIL/7/2177, Collection 48/36 Dr A.D. Mackinnon to Mr Jackson, memo, 13 April 1895; BL IOR/L/MIL/7/14471, Collection 323/49 Medical Subordinates for Service in East Africa, letter, 28 January 1907

28 *AMR*, 1921, p. 21

29 BL IOR/MIL/7/2177 Collection 48/25 Uganda Railway, Memo to Lord Hamilton, Secretary of State, 11 March 1896; John Iliffe states that MOs got two or three times

higher pay than Assistant Surgeons. Iliffe, *East African Doctors*, p. 78. For European MO salaries see Crozier, *Practising Colonial Medicine*, pp. 27–8

30   BL IOR/MIL/7/2177 Memo to Lord Hamilton, 11 March 1896; BL IOR/L/MIL/7/14626 Collection 324A/122,COD No 855: Revised Rules for the Employment of Assistant Surgeons and Compounders in the British East Africa and Uganda Protectorates Recruited from Sources Outside of the Service of the Government of India, 9 November 1917

31   For the necessity to make economic savings through retrenchments see Gilks, 'The Medical Department', p. 350

32   It proved frustrating to reconcile the staffing figures variously presented in *The Medical Register of the Official Gazette of the East Africa Protectorate* (after 1920 *The Official Gazette of the Kenya Government*), *The Medical Department Annual Medical Reports*, *The Medical Directory* and the Colonial Office 'Blue Books'. All four sources slightly differently defined what 'medical staff' constituted and not all held information for all periods. For consistency, this study uses the figures given in the *AMR* each year (aside from 1903, when no *AMR* was available, so the Blue Book was used).

33   Although some accounts do exist. See RHL Papers Collected by H. Topiwala Related to Indian Doctors in Kenya, expected deposit date 2015 (although this documents the experiences of private doctors, there were undoubtedly some similarities with Indian government doctors in terms of the socio-medical worlds they faced); district medical reports are also very useful (see below, note 33). Very early experiences are recorded in BL IOR/L/MIL/7/12673, H.D. Masani, Report on the Health of the Mombasa Force, including 24th Bombay Infantry, 3 June 1896 and BL IOR/MIL/7/14462: 1899–1901, Collection 323/40 Promotion of Uganda Railway Hospital Assistant Rahmat Ali, which records a rare personal story.

34   RHL MSS.Afr.s.702 Robert Arthur Welsford Procter, 'Random Reminiscences, Mainly Surgical' [no date]; Crozier, *Practising Colonial Medicine*, pp. 87–8

35   Syracuse University (SU), Kenya National Archive Records (KNA), Microfilm Number 2801, Annual and Quarterly Reports (Provincial and District) Reel 15: Provincial Medical Report, E.B. Horne, Meru, 1915 and 1916; Provincial Medical Report, Abdulla Khan, Meru, 1918–20; Provincial Medical Report, Ali Baksh, Meru, 1922; Reel 21: Provincial Medical Report, Gokul Chand, Kabarnet, 1921; Reel 56: Provincial Medical Report Maula Buksh, Kilifi, 1918–19; Reel 59: Provincial Medical Reports, Maula Buksh, Malindi, 1918–19

36   A.N. Nyss, *AMR*, 1919, p. 14; *AMR*, 1921, p. 22

37   SU KNA Microfilm Number 2801, Annual and Quarterly Reports (Provincial and District), Reel 21: Provincial Medical Report, Gokul Chand, Kabarnet, 1921, Provincial and District Reports, Gokul Chand, Kabarnet Medical Report, p. 30; See also: Wellcome Library, Contemporary Medical Archives Centre, PP/HCT/A5 Elizabeth Bray, 'Hugh Trowell: Pioneer Nutritionist', unpublished biography, London 1988

38   A.N. Nyss, *AMR*, 1913, pp. 77–80

39   T.D. Nair, 'A Tana River Yaws Campaign', *Kenya and East Africa Medical Journal*, 1927, pp. 201–7

40   Salvadori, *We Came in Dhows*, vol. 3, p. 140

41   SU KNA Microfilm Number 2801, Annual and Quarterly Reports (Provincial and District) Reel 15: Provincial Medical Report, E.B. Horne, Meru, 1915 and 1916; Provincial Medical Report, Abdulla Khan, Meru, 1918–20

42   SU KNA Microfilm Number 2801, Annual and Quarterly Reports (Provincial and District) Reel 21: Provincial Medical Report, Gokul Chand, Kabarnet, 1921

43   SU KNA Microfilm Number 2801, Annual and Quarterly Reports (Provincial and District) Reel 21: Provincial Medical Report, Gokul Chand, Kabarnet, 1921

44   Milne, 'The Rise of the Colonial Medical Service', p. 58

45   Milne, 'The Rise of the Colonial Medical Service', p. 58

46   RHL MSS.Afr.s.1872/75 Robert Samuel Hennessey, 'Memorandum on Experiences in the Colonial Medical Service in Uganda, 1929–55'

47   RHL MSS.Brit.Emp.r.4 Peter Alphonsus Clearkin, 'Ramblings and Recollections of a Colonial Doctor 1913–58', Book I, Durban, 1967, typescript, p. 126
48   BL IOR/L/PJ/6/1718 *Economic Commission Report 1919*, Nairobi, Swift Press, 1919, pp. 20–1
49   Ethel Younghusband, *Glimpses of East Africa and Zanzibar*, London, John Long, 1910, p. 219
50   'Mass Meeting and Dr Burkitt', *East African Chronicle*, 13 August 1921, pp. 4, 8, 9
51   'Hardinge's Administrative Proposals, 6 July 1895', in G.H. Mungeam, *Kenya: Select Historical Documents 1884–1923*, Nairobi, East African Publishing House, 1979, pp. 69–75
52   M.P.K. Sorrenson, *Origin of European Settlement in Kenya*, London, Oxford University Press, 1968, p. 34
53   Charles Eliot, 1905, quoted in Gregory, *India and East Africa*, p. 46
54   Bruce Berman and John Lonsdale, *Unhappy Valley: Conflict in Kenya and Africa, Book 1: State and Class*, London, James Currey, 1991, p. 34; B.M. Du Toit, *The Boers in East Africa: Ethnicity and Identity*, London, Bergen and Garvey, 1998, p. 24; C.S. Nichols, *Red Strangers: The White Tribes of Kenya*, London, Timewell Press, 2005, p. 49
55   Diana Wylie, 'Confrontation over Kenya: The Colonial Office and Its Critics, 1918–1940', *Journal of African History*, 18,3, 1977, pp. 427–47, at p. 445
56   Mangat, *History of the Asians in East Africa*, pp. 97–131. R.M. Maxon, *Struggle for Kenya: The Loss and Reassertion of Imperial Initiative, 1912–1923*, London, Fairleigh Dickinson University Press, 1993, pp. 52, 111
57   Keith Kyle, 'Gandhi, Harry Thuku and Early Kenya Nationalism', *Transition*, 27, 1966, pp. 16–22, at p. 17; Robert J. Blyth, *The Empire of the Raj: India, Eastern Africa and the Middle East, 1858–1947*, Cambridge, Cambridge University Press, 2003, pp. 104–19
58   BL IOR/L/PJ/6/1718 *Economic Commission Report 1919*, Nairobi, Swift Press, 1919, p. 21
59   BL IOR/L/PJ/6/1718 *Economic Commission Report 1919*, Nairobi, Swift Press, 1919, p. 21
60   BL IOR/L/PJ/6/1718 *Economic Commission Report 1919*, Nairobi, Swift Press, 1919, p. 21
61   Edward Paice, *Lost Lion of Empire: The Life of 'Cape to Cairo' Grogan*, London, Harper Collins, 2001, pp. 291, 450
62   TNA CO/544/29, Kenya Legislative Council Minutes, 3 January 1922; re proposal to set up the Committee, see W.G. Ross, *Kenya from Within: A Short Political History*, London, George Allen, 1927, pp. 159–60. See also Delamere's representation to Churchill regarding the high cost of Asian clerks and medical staff in the absence of trained African staff: TNA CO/533/451/2 memorandum 14 February 1922 on colonial expenditure. Information on the proposed 20% reduction can be found in: Anon, 'Asiatics Salaries Cut: Indian Reply to Geddes Committee Suggestion', *The Leader*, 20 May 1922, p. 8
63   TNA CO/544/29 B.S. Varma, Minutes of the Kenya Legislative Council, 22 October 1922
64   BL IOR/L/E/7/1264 The Devonshire Declaration, White Paper, Cmd 1922
65   Christopher P. Youé, 'The Threat of Settler Rebellion and the Imperial Predicament: The Denial of Indian Rights in Kenya, 1923', *Canadian Journal of History*, 12, 1978, pp. 347–60; Blyth, *Empire of the Raj*, pp. 93–131; Randolph M.K. Joalahliae, *The Indian as an Enemy: An Analysis of the Indian Question in East Africa*, Bloomington, IN, Authorhouse, 2010; Sana Aiyar, 'Empire, Race and the Indians in Colonial Kenya's Contested Public Political Sphere, 1919–1923', *Africa: The Journal of the International African Institute*, 81, 1, 2011, pp. 132–54
66   *AMR*, 1913, p. 18
67   W.J. Simpson, *Report on the Sanitary Matters in the East African Protectorate, Uganda and Zanzibar*, London, Colonial Office, Africa No. 1025, 1915, pp. 9–10
68   Simpson, *Report on Sanitary Matters*, 1915, pp. 9–10

69   The most important concerned: Epidemic Control (1902), Infectious Diseases (1903), Sleeping Sickness (1903), Plague and Cholera (1907), Vaccination (1912), Mosquito and Malaria in Townships (1912) and Quarantine (1913).

70   BL IOR/L/E/7/1265 Winston Churchill, memorandum, 29 April 1921. For the discussion of clause 15 in the Kenya Legislative Council see *The Leader*, 29 January 1921, p. 3

71   TNA CO/533/394/1 Racial Segregation in Towns, memorandum, 25 March 1931

72   Peter Clearkin described Gilks as having the 'great weakness of trying to curry favours with settlers or their hangers on', RHL MSS.Brit.Emp.r.4 Peter Alphonsus Clearkin, 'Ramblings and Recollections of a Colonial Doctor 1913–58', Book II, Durban, 1967, typescript, p. 162; See also TNA CO/544/29 Kenya Legislative Council Minutes 1921–29, Debate on the Medical Department, 29 October 1923, when Varma, the Indian member, proposed an unsuccessful motion to reduce Gilks's salary by £100 to emphasise that Indian and African communities were not served well by him.

73   TNA CO/544/29, Kenya Legislative Council Minutes, 24 January 1921; TNA CO/544/14 Kenya Executive Council Minutes, 7 May 1921, pp. 640, 761; BL IOR/E/7/1265 [unidentified newspaper cutting on Gilks's change of heart over the segregation clause], 29 January 1921

74   Our parenthesis. TNA CO/544/29 Kenya Legislative Council Minutes, 27 March 1922

75   *AMR*, 1921 p. 18; *AMR*, 1923, p. 1

76   British Medical Association Archive (BMA) B/162/1/9, BMA Dominions Committee Documents, Session 1921–22, Meeting 30 June 1922, p. 1

77   BMA B/162/1/12 Dominions Committee Documents, Session 1924–5, 6 March 1925, p. 3; Memorandum on Medical and Sanitary Services from Kenya BMA Branch, 5 March 1925

78   *AMR*, 1924, p. 1; Iliffe, *East African Doctors*, p. 24

79   *AMR*, 1936, p. 7

80   *AMR*, 1932, p. 2. The others could have been nurses (confusingly called Hospital Assistants), but also in other junior roles, such as orderlies, storekeepers, clerks gardeners, sweepers etc. The competence of African dressers was sometimes praised in the official *AMRs* but the judgement was contradicted in the PMOs' own internal memos (e.g. TNA CO/533/426/8 Native Medical Service, 1932), which were highly critical.

81   *AMR*, 1937, p. 7, Table III

82   See note 31 above.

83   Beck, *A History of the British Medical Administration*; Crozier, *Practising Colonial Medicine*

84   But, interestingly, all the studies of middle-level healthcare workers have been of black Africans. See, for example, Anne Digby, 'The Mid-Level Health Worker in South Africa: The In-Between Condition of the "Middle"', in Ryan Johnson and Amna Khalid (eds.), *Public Health in the British Empire: Intermediaries, Subordinates, and the Practice of Public Health*, New York and London, Routledge, 2012, pp. 171–92. See also the discussion in Marku Hokkanen, *Medicine and Scottish Missionaries in the Northern Malawi Region, 1875–1930*, Lampeter, Edwin Mellen Press, 2007, pp. 412–20

85   Adeloya Adeloye, *African Pioneers of Modern Medicine: Nigerian Doctors of the Nineteenth Century*, Ibadan, University Press Limited, 1985; Adell Patton, *Physicians, Colonial Racism and Diaspora in West Africa*, Gainesville, FL, University of Florida Press, 1996; Iliffe, *East African Doctors*; Anne Digby, 'Early Black Doctors in South Africa', *Journal of African History*, 46, 2005, pp. 427–54

86   For a fuller, book-length exploration of this history of Indian doctors, including GPs, in Kenya see: Anna Greenwood and Harshad Topiwala, *Indian Doctors in Kenya: The Forgotten Story, 1895–1940*, London, Palgrave Macmillan, 2015

CHAPTER FIVE

The Colonial Medical Service and the struggle for control of the Zanzibar Maternity Association, 1918–47

Anna Greenwood

British colonialists on Zanzibar frequently grumbled that its colourful demographic character was a particular headache to their administration. When the British formally established their administration in 1890 they encountered a 'distinctly urban, mercantile and cosmopolitan' island economy which had developed over centuries and was headed by Sultan Sayyid Ali bin Said Al-Busaid and his extravagant court.[1] Zanzibar was home to a thriving merchant class of Arabs and Indians, as well as poorer members of these communities, co-existing alongside the majority African poor.[2] Even British generalisations had to concede that this was far from the supposed blank canvas implied through rhetorical representations of the mainland Dark Continent.[3] Forced to be sensitive to the existing political structures, the British ruled Zanzibar as a protected Arab state, leaving the Sultan as constitutional head until 1913 (and indeed as a figurehead until independence in 1963). Furthermore, they adapted their administration to the existing hierarchies on the island by retaining the Arab ruling caste and by staffing the lower ranks of their administration with 'mudirs' – members of the local Arab elite – who acted in a similar role to British District Officers on the mainland.[4] Despite its proximity to the African mainland, Zanzibar's distinctiveness was pronounced and it was regarded as given that it needed special and relatively subtle political management. This region was, according to one contemporary commentator, a 'huddled, unplanned block of Asia', where life was 'not African' and the ancient capital, Stone Town, was '[e]ssentially ... an Arab town'.[5]

Although Zanzibar was defined as one set of islands, it contained various well-established communities. Most were comprised of Africans of Bantu origin, but these were increasingly joined by Africans of various ethnic groups from the mainland. The next biggest group were immigrants from Arabia, principally from Muscat, Oman or

Hadramaut. A further section of the population had ties to the Indian subcontinent, made up of Indians, Pakistanis and Goans – a religious mix of Moslems, Ismailis and Hindus. The situation presents a striking historical example of a colonial power having to formulate policies that were applicable to different, yet cohabiting, populations.

The ethnic diversity of the island posed particular challenges for the British medical authorities. Despite acting as the main quarantine station for Kenya, Tanganyika and Uganda, the hub of Stone Town was renowned for its disease-ridden port and overpowering stench. The islands were nicknamed 'Stinkibar' by David Livingstone in 1866, leading to routine associations with a whole gamut of public health problems.[6] British medical control was hindered by the perplexing range of indigenous behaviour towards matters of health, making any blanket public health policy frustratingly difficult to conceive, apply and police. In Zanzibar 'Africa, Arabia and Asia seem to meet and blend', bemoaned one medical commentator in 1924, directly creating 'all kinds of sanitary questions … in consequence'.[7]

The case of the Zanzibar Maternity Association (ZMA) provides one example of the British negotiation of this racial diversity on Zanzibar. By showing that the Colonial Medical Service was increasingly unhappy to work with another healthcare provider on Zanzibar – in this case the majority Indian- and Arab-funded ZMA – we are given an instructive lens through which to examine the way colonial medical policy was sometimes selectively deployed. This shows, above all, how the British sought to manipulate their self-image in relation to the racial politics of the island, in ways that flexibly prioritised their own interests.

Despite the fact that that the ZMA had originally been a British idea, and irrespective of the Association's subsequent popularity and success, the Colonial Medical Service showed itself to be uninterested in supporting medical initiatives unless it was allowed to fully control and manage them. Although the ZMA filled a conspicuous gap within the healthcare provision offered by the Colonial Medical Service on Zanzibar, the British government was happy to fund and cooperate with it only if it could essentially run it as an adjunct part of the colonial medical department. When the Arab and Indian funders objected to this – at least wanting credit for their initiatives – the British were quick to disparage the ZMA and the recipients of its services, often in quite strong language. Surprisingly, the British eschewed, rather than embraced, the opportunity of working with rich local philanthropists, notwithstanding the potential of the situation to promote the magnanimity and cooperativeness of British imperial overlordship.

While the focus of this chapter is a maternity association, the issue is not birthing practices, or the development of colonial maternal health policy as such – this has been extensively explored in other writings about Empire.[8] Rather, this example is chosen as an illustration of the way the Colonial Medical Service could be sometimes mistrustful about working beyond what it felt to constitute the remit of the State, whether that be with missionary clinics, schools or local charitable initiatives. The story of the tumultuous British relations with the ZMA illustrates how uneasy the British were about being eclipsed or even simply not credited with being the most important givers of formal medical care on the island. As the ZMA was supported mostly through Indian and Arab coffers, the British were nervous about the service the ZMA provided, even though they had no alternative government maternity care provision of their own to offer and even though the model of maternity care provided by the ZMA was broadly in accordance with Western biomedical principles in so far as it advocated precepts of Western hygiene and promoted the benefits of hospital care in some circumstances.

The case of the ZMA also shows how the British were prepared to elastically deploy racial arguments against their Indian and Arab colonial subjects to suit their needs. While in some situations it was regarded as appropriate to work with locals (for example by employing mudirs, or employing Indian Assistant and Sub-Assistant Surgeons within the colonial medical department; see Chapter Four), equally there were situations when cooperation was evidently deemed less desirable.[9] The essential point seemed to be the necessity of decisive government control. If the Indians, Arabs or Africans were employed by the colonial state, even in relatively influential roles, the dominance of the British seemed safe. To cooperate with these groups on a more equal footing, particularly when they were the majority funders of an enterprise and argued for proportionate influence in its affairs – as was the case with the ZMA – was far less desirable.

This example highlights a rarely discussed area of colonial governance, although it ultimately makes no firm conclusion as to whether racial politics were an epiphenomenon or a determinant of colonial policy. What it does usefully show, however, is that while it is now universally accepted that the British were racist in their attitudes and actions towards their colonial subjects, also these attitudes could be subtly and selectively deployed adaptively and responsively to local situations. In colonial Africa, Africans were habitually portrayed as the least civilised race, the lowest rung in the racial hierarchy. But, as the case of the ZMA shows, when it suited their aims, the British characterised Indians and Arabs as far worse than the Africans, pinpointing them as the most primitive ethnic groups on the island and in need of reform.[10] Indeed, ZMA archive files show that, where expedient, Africans were often praised as showing openness to change and reform, in contrast to the intransigent attitudes of their Indian and Arab counterparts.

One of the reasons put forward by the British as to why they were unhappy to support the ZMA was that members of the Arab and Indian communities principally claimed its services. This is intriguing. Although the ethnic diversity of Zanzibar had been established over centuries, and was acknowledged by the British in many of their other policies (such as the decision to allow Islamic law to function in tandem with colonial law on Zanzibar), somehow the British still felt that it was acceptable to insinuate that their medical services were principally directed at just *some* of their colonial subjects. In short, by complaining about the way the ZMA principally helped Indian and Arab communities, the British seemed to be implying that they held a preference to help black Africans, rather than the members of the Indian or Arab community. The reason for this seems evident: Indians and Arabs were perceived as providing the most tangible threats to British superiority. In the case of the struggles over the control over the ZMA it therefore suited Colonial Medical Service objectives to portray Indians and Arabs as untrustworthy sponsors – representatives of communities that were particularly susceptible to disease and that lacked personal hygiene.

The Zanzibar Maternity Association and the British

The ZMA was a quasi-autonomous charity founded in 1918 on the advice of three British officials, two of whom were government doctors: Mr Crofton, Dr Copland and Dr Curwen. The organisation was conceived as a means of supplying trained midwives to attend Asiatic, Arab and African women in their confinements. Although ZMA services briefly expanded to outlying rural areas in the early 1930s, these were never very successful and the ZMA principally catered for the multi-ethnic inhabitants of Zanzibar's thriving capital, known as Stone Town. As registrations of births on Zanzibar were unreliable, it is difficult to gauge how successful the ZMA was in real terms, although the yearly statistics show that attendances rose steadily throughout its existence, except for a dip in 1933, which was explained away as part of the worldwide Depression.[11] The high point of its success was achieved in 1938, when as many as 75 per cent of all births taking place in Zanzibar Town were attended by ZMA midwives.[12] An important feature of the service was that it did not insist on hospital care for expectant mothers and also aimed to provide culturally relevant services for the communities of Zanzibar Town via home visits.[13]

From the start the ZMA had a rather ambiguous status. It had been a British idea, but it was declared by a government officer as 'a private enterprise ... [without] the same permanence as a Government undertaking'.[14] Crucially, it was not considered part of official colonial medical policy – to the extent that the founding of the ZMA was not mentioned in the government Annual Medical Report (AMR).[15] While it was described as 'not a Government institution' it was also said to be 'under the Patronage of the Zanzibar Government', with the terms left sufficiently vague to allow the interpretation that both the British colonial government and the hereditary sultanate, which was also a patron of Association activities, had joint responsibility.[16] Although ZMA leadership always comprised a British (often non-medical) official,[17] it was not absorbed into the British colonial administration until 1947, principally because its reliance on external patronage would have been at risk if the British assumed dominance.

The British contributed an annual grant (initially 4,500 rupees[18]) towards the running of the ZMA and the rest of the Association was supported by private subscriptions and donations, as well as from the profits made from any fees charged to patients who could afford to pay (set at 75 shillings per case).[19] Particularly prominent in funding the ZMA was the Wakf Commission (based on the ancient Islamic law of *waqf*), which oversaw the spending of Islamic endowments for the purposes of charity.[20] This Commission was set up on Zanzibar by the British in 1905 to oversee the distribution of wakf, so this contribution was sanctioned by the British even if its sources were not British.[21] Also highly significant in the funding profile were Tharia Topan, who controlled and distributed the inheritance of his forebear, the knighted Ismaili Indian merchant and Zanzibari philanthropist of the same name; and the Indian National Association, which paid for beds to be made available for Association mothers in the Mkunazini Hospital (in the days before the ZMA had its own hospital facility) and also paid the salary of the ZMA's European midwife, Miss Locket.[22] From its inauguration, the different funding bodies represented in the ZMA's quarterly meeting General Committee struggled to gain ascendancy and to stipulate the ZMA's agenda. While the Indian and Arab representatives understandably wanted to make provision for their own communities, the British tended to advance the African cause, which they increasingly saw as their responsibility within the terms of the dual mandate.

Aside from the date of its foundation, a few other dates mark important points in the history of the ZMA and highlight the progressively acrimonious relations that developed between the Association and the Colonial Medical Service and peaked during the 1930s. In 1925 the

Mwembeladu Maternity Home was opened as the institutional base for maternal welfare work. The home, 'built largely from funds provided by the Tharia Topan family',[23] was also substantially funded (30,000 rupees (Rs)) by the Wakf Commission, with the internal furniture and fittings provided by the prominent Indian company Messrs Karimjee Jivanjee and Co.[24] Although the British government was not the primary funder of this home, it did increase its annual grant to the ZMA from Rs 4,500 to Rs 7,500 when it opened, and agreed to supply free drugs and dressings for its patients. The first decade of Mwembeladu's existence, however, was characterised by struggles over its control and marked the beginnings of the distinct souring of relations between the British government and the ZMA.[25] When the home opened in 1925 the British had assumed that it would be under the control of their medical department,[26] but the majority members of the ZMA, who had secured funding for the building and its contents, naturally envisaged it as independent of British state control. By 1934 intransience by members of the ZMA on this issue meant that the British had to concede that 'what little control government had in the past has now been lost', and in 1937 the control of Mwembeladu was officially declared as being solely back in ZMA hands.[27] This decisive move underlined ZMA preferences for independence and was conducted as part of a broader revision of the structure and remit of the ZMA, resulting in the new Reserved Articles of the Association of 1937.[28]

A period of particularly intense British criticism led up to this 1937 administrative overhaul. In 1932 the ZMA announced its hope to start a midwife-training programme, as a means of extending its services to the rural areas. It planned to recruit rural women for training at Mwembeladu and then let them return to their home communities to practise their skills.[29] This scheme got off the ground in 1933 with the opening of seven rural centres, but it soon became apparent that the problems of the Depression and limited funding meant that the initiative was not viable unless external contributions could be found. The British, however, refused to help the ZMA in their scheme, a move which ensured its failure.[30] Without British support, the ZMA had no option but to hand control over to the government, which promptly reversed its earlier opposition to the scheme and offered to take it over entirely from 1935.[31] Immediately upon taking control, however, the medical department embarked upon a regional survey, damningly concluding that it was 'unfavourably impressed by these rural centres' and recommending that all but one should be closed down.[32] To add insult to injury, the British government then announced that, as compensation for taking over the centre work from the Association, it would reduce its grant to the ZMA by Rs 600 a year, despite its intention to close down most of the newly acquired rural centres.[33] This episode provides a striking example of the way the British used the financial pressures of the ZMA for their own advantage. They knew that the ZMA could not expand without their support and went so far as to financially punish the ZMA for its apparent lack of foresight. The bitter attitude of the British medical department preferred total absence of rural maternity services to exclusive provision by the ZMA.

Concurrently with this crisis in relations – and not entirely unconnected to it – there occurred a period of separate 'quarrels' between the ZMA and the British administration about the 'misapplication of funds' and arguments about 'general control and representation on the committee'.[34] Particular attention was paid in these arguments to the dominant role played in the ZMA General Committee by Tharia Topan. The British government declared that it felt as if it had had 'a pistol held to its head by Tharia Topan' since his appointment to the committee in 1928,[35] because 'he felt he should have a larger say in matters concerning the Association than other members of the Committee'.[36] British dissatisfaction with Topan was so recurrent that eventually the ZMA, faced with the threat of alienating British funding altogether, was forced to negotiate a compromise with him, securing his retirement from their governing board.[37]

The 1937 new Reserved Articles of the Association were produced in reaction to this dissatisfaction over representation, financial mismanagement and long-brewing misunderstandings over administrative proprietorship of the Mwembeladu Home. The aim was to make the ZMA more transparent and administratively efficient and was a clear response to vocal British claims of financial incompetence, cumbersome bureaucracy and internal discord.[38] Superficially, this bureaucratic clarification looked like an attempt to establish the charity's independence from the British government. Although British officials still presided on the committee, and the British government still financially contributed to its affairs, the ZMA officially declared itself to be 'no-longer under the control of the Medical Department and managed by its own committee'.[39]

In effect, this was to be the ZMA's final assertion of defiance and independence. Almost as soon as the Articles were enacted, the British began to actively pursue investigations into the financial dealings of the ZMA and to re-agitate for control over Mwembeladu. In 1939 direct accusations were made against the ZMA by the new colonial Medical Officer in charge, Dr Sydney Lee. Lee declared that ZMA funds for Mwembeladu were internally mismanaged, and also called into question the government's historic agreement with the ZMA to supply free drugs and dressings to the home.[40] Outside the ZMA committee,

Association members were suspicious of Lee's investigations, declaring that his actions were intended 'to prove that the government should take over the Home by bringing the Association into some disrepute'.[41] Rumours circulated that 'there was little secrecy about the hope or intention of the Medical Department to take over this home'.[42]

These prolonged investigations coincided with more general moves towards the regulation of colonial midwifery. The British government seized upon them as further support for its argument that the ZMA could function adequately only if it was run and policed by the Colonial Medical Service. The Central Midwives Board in the UK had been established in 1902, but during the 1940s it began to extend its regulatory framework for the training and conduct of midwives within the British Empire. Partly in response to this, in 1942 Medical Officer Violet Sharp introduced her new formal training scheme for midwives on Zanzibar – a clear snub to ZMA midwifery training initiatives which had been underway since the 1930s. Miss Locket, the ZMA chief midwife, was only too aware that tighter restrictions were to be introduced and saw the potential effects that this would have on the ZMA, which relied on illiterate local midwives trained via an apprenticeship system. Locket anxiously wrote to the ZMA president in 1943 that 'everything has now been completely changed', owing to the new provisions instituted by the Central Midwives Board in the UK, which were soon to be rolled out to the colonies.[43] In effect, the British used their colonial power to undermine ZMA midwifery training activities by pointing out that they did not comply with international standards.

The succession of events was relatively rapid. By 1944 discussions were already underway for the ZMA presidency to be taken over by a British Medical Officer, and in 1947 – the year of Indian independence and a point when nervousness about colonial rule was at a high – the British government formally took over control of the ZMA, installing Dr J.C. Earl as president and severely limiting Indian and Arab representation. Significantly, Earl's first act as was to enact his Midwives Decree (no. 12) 1945, which he had personally drawn up himself, finally formalising midwifery provision and training on Zanzibar in accordance with British guidelines and standards.[44] Tellingly, the British ultimately referred to colonial law and governance as their final lever to justify their dominance over the ZMA. Insistence that the ZMA's practices and training provision were not in accord with the stipulations of the British government as enshrined in the Central Midwives Board was the most powerful means by which the government could exert pressure on the ZMA. Against such legislative pressures, the ZMA had little option other than to capitulate.

Maternal health on Zanzibar

The work of the ZMA and the tensions between it and the British government need to be understood in the broader context of colonial maternal health provision at that time. It is striking that the Colonial Medical Service was so antagonistic towards the ZMA, as no other formal provision for maternal welfare existed in Zanzibar under the government medical services. As the government itself admitted in 1928: '[b]eyond rendering all possible assistance to the Zanzibar Maternity Association, the Government medical staff has little time to give to this important branch of public health work'.[45] The ZMA provided the only organised maternal welfare work in the region, and yet the British were increasingly unprepared to cooperate with it. Over and beyond the local tensions, this perhaps demonstrated a more general nervousness about any organised social provision on the island outside government control.

The late arrival of government maternal and child welfare services in Zanzibar is somewhat of an anomaly in the region. This was partly because of Zanzibar's island status, which meant that, despite its strategic importance as the main port of entry for East and Central Africa, the Colonial Office tended to channel financial and personnel resources into its larger, more politically prominent territories on the mainland. Medical reports of the period all reiterated the ill-effects of the chronic lack of resources and constantly complained about the lack of personnel and the consequent inability to make any real inroads into either hospital-based or community-based healthcare provision. The low priority afforded to maternal healthcare on Zanzibar (no mention was made of maternal or child health in any AMR before 1922[46]) should be understood in this local context, but it was still enormously behind the rest of Empire; with discussions of colonial healthcare within contemporary textbooks devoting chapters to the centrality of structured maternity care within British possessions.[47] In fact, maternity and child health within the colonies increasingly became a key topic for discussion from the interwar years onwards, reflecting similar preoccupations in the domestic sphere in Britain.[48]

Indeed, the lack of such healthcare provision on Zanzibar also frustrated the British medical administration. It was conventional throughout Empire for a Woman Medical Officer (WMO) to be appointed to oversee maternity and child welfare work and, from 1924, the British medical department on Zanzibar regularly lobbied the Colonial Office to have such a colonial servant posted to the island.[49] It took twelve years, however, before Dr Violet Sharp was finally appointed in May 1936,[50] twenty-five years after Uganda, where the WMO position had been filled in 1911.[51] The Zanzibar Director of Medical Services, Leslie Webb, retrospectively explained away this discrepancy as being due to the comparative 'urgency' of the situation in Uganda, where syphilis was widespread, whereas the disease did 'not appear to be a major problem' in Zanzibar.[52]

Unsurprisingly, Dr Sharp's arrival did not bring any immediate change to the state of official maternal healthcare provision. When the chief medical advisor to the colonial officer, A.J.R. O'Brien, visited Zanzibar in 1938, he announced that he was 'displeased to find that Government undertook so little maternity work'. He also expressed his alarm at the ZMA arrangements at Mwembeladu Maternity Home. How could it be that the home was 'controlled by a Committee of 10 Indians or Goans, 3 Arabs, 1 African and 1 European' and yet had 'all expenses ... borne by the government'?[53] This complaint neatly encapsulates the fundamental anxieties of the British government. Although the British were unable to offer any alternative organised maternity provision on Zanzibar until the early 1940s, they were nevertheless extremely anxious about the work of the ZMA and what this might indicate in terms of the erosion of (their perceived) Western medical hegemony. Simply put, the medical department found it very difficult to support any healthcare facility that it could not absolutely control, regardless of the local needs it fulfilled or the popularity it enjoyed.

Health discourses and Colonial Medical Service complaints about the ZMA

At the heart of the increasingly problematic relations between the ZMA and the Colonial Medical Service lay the general assumption of European racial superiority, as demonstrated throughout Empire in the motives of the civilising mission. This construed the British role to educate and to reform indigenous populations and, in matters of health, paid particular attention to the alleged lack of hygiene and particular propensities towards disease of the 'unreformed' and pathological indigenes; a tendency which has been explored at length within the colonial medical literature.[54] Quite naturally the Colonial Medical Service's attitudes on Zanzibar conformed to this general model, with medical reports frequently bemoaning that no amount of help or external improvements in matters of health would help indigenous people (including, in the context of Zanzibar, Arabs and Indians) if they were not prepared to help themselves. A short history of the ZMA, written by an anonymous British official, explicitly reminisced on the regrettable predominance of old-fashioned birthing practices that existed in 1918:

> Prior to its inception the populace was dependent on the services of untrained and ignorant women whose unclean habits and ingrained prejudices and customs were responsible for much suffering and mortality among lying-in women and new-born children.[55]

Typically, high mortality and propensity towards disease were explained in terms of indigenous culpability through resistance to change. Similarly, the 1927 AMR of the British government declared that:

> Natives of a tropical country have many and varied parasites to contend with. Their past traditions are those of apathy and indifference and these can only be gradually overcome. Nothing dramatic can therefore be expected, but rather a gradual improvement spread over the course of years.[56]

Ideas specifically connecting maternal health with flawed and unhygienic behaviour were particularly marked. The need for maternal health provision was presented as one of the most important challenges because indigenous women were generally considered to be especially superstitious influences within the social fabric. As one medical report warned: '[t]he women to a much greater extent than the men are imbued with superstition and it is they who insist on charms and incantations and delay calling in skilled medical assistance until too late'.[57] The declared purpose of the ZMA was to offer a modern alternative to traditional models of maternal health, counteracting, for example, the influence of:

> untrained *dayas* whose ignorance, prejudices and unhygienic methods were responsible for much suffering and mortality amongst lying-in women and new-born children. Shocking stories were current of methods employed. [Dr] Curwen told me of a case in which a piece of rope was tied round the neck of a half-born baby and a stone attached to aid delivery.[58]

The self-proclaimed ardency of the ZMA to bring clean and safe modern practices to traditional communities gave it an affinity with the biomedical priorities of the Colonial Medical Service, which was also preoccupied with stamping out superstition and enlightening its colonial subjects to the benefits of modern Western medical techniques. However, during times of conflict between the two groups, the British preferred to distance themselves from the funders of the ZMA, often making derogatory comments against the health habits and management acumen of the Indian, and, most damningly, the Arab, populations of Zanzibar. Such negative rhetoric was used to justify attitudes towards, and even sanctions against, these particular groups.[59] These colonial discourses were intriguingly out of kilter with customary racial generalisations, which tended to place the influential Arab and

Indian elite far higher than Africans in terms of social status – indeed the Arabs themselves were keen to stress the huge gulf between their 'civilised' Islamic culture and the 'barbarous' African one.[60] British files on the ZMA reveal that racial stereotypes were applied rather flexibly (within the overall paradigm of European superiority) to suit the circumstances presented by different colonial situations.

The ZMA management stressed that the Association did not 'confine its activities to any one sect' and was a 'social service non-racial in character', but conflicts about racial priorities nonetheless permeate internal struggles over its remit during the 1930s.[61] As the Association was mainly funded from Indian and Arab sources, it was primarily concerned with helping mothers within these local communities; certainly they were by the far the largest groups cited in the ZMA's annual reports as using its midwives.[62] Even this provision was sometimes contested, however, with various religious and ethnic subgroups of the Arab and Indian communities sporadically complaining that funds were not being targeted at the specific communities for which they had been intended.[63] Theoretically at least, the ZMA was supposed to be equally committed to helping Africans, and the apparent lack of even-handedness in pursuing this point (not entirely borne out by the figures, which showed gradually increasing African attendances[64]) was the one which the British seized upon and repeatedly used to denounce the ZMA for its bias in favour of the Arab and Indian communities of Zanzibar Town.[65]

At the same time, the British frequently used opportunities to criticise the health habits of the Arab and Indian communities, characterising them as far from redemption in matters of health and hygiene, and hence calling into question the utility and effectiveness of the ZMA. This was an inversion of the usual British ordering of indigenous civilisations, but it crucially served British purposes in that it tarnished the reputation of the group that was giving the government the most competition (with all the implied political threats that this entailed) on the islands. A snippet from the *AMR 1921* is indicative:

> It is to be regretted that the average poor-class Indian is utterly deficient in any sense of hygiene. To shut out all light and air, to crowd together, to spit freely and constantly all over the place, whether indoors or out, seem to be ingrained habits with them. They have a complete disregard of sanitation laws for the public welfare and are quite prepared to hide cases of infectious disease if they think that its notification to the authorities will cause them inconvenience, as was shown in the case of Small-pox concealed by Indians in the bazaars. The natives, too, are equally fond of stuffiness, overcrowding and expectoration, and, although when they live in their own mud and wattle huts *they make*

some attempt at cleanliness, they soon lose this when they crowd into the already crowded bazaars.[66]

A similar conclusion was reached in an assessment of the health and hygiene of school children: '[a]s regards cleanliness, there is no doubt that the Africans and Comorians are the cleanest, and the Arabs are cleaner than the Indians'. The British medical author went on to specify that '[d]efects of vision are commonest in Indians and Arabs, as are defective teeth'.[67] Time and again the same negative rhetoric related matters of poor hygiene, with the 'Arab, Shihiri and Comoro communities' claiming them to be 'the most backward in realizing the benefits of Western methods'.[68]

It might be thought that if the British genuinely felt that the Arab and Indian communities of Zanzibar were most in need of health improvements, these sectors would be thought the most deserving – or at least the most worthy targets of reform – but rather, the British seemed to use these denunciatory images to justify and help reiterate their exclusive orientation towards the African communities. This points to the crux of the issue, clearly summarised in a letter of 1942:

> [The] Government is primarily concerned with the training of African Midwives for work in rural areas amongst Africans; whereas the Association is concerned primarily in providing a Town service for Indian and Arab people, though naturally the services of the Association's midwives are not denied to Africans. The Association [therefore] caters for an unavoidable Racial [*sic* capitalisation] prejudice ...[69]

If the British were going to help indigenous groups via their medical department (as was becoming the colonial expectation by the 1920s), they wanted to be seen to be helping Africans. This emphasis was quite explicit. From the time the ZMA was founded in 1918 the British government made it clear that its proportion of the ZMA grant was only 'intended to cover free treatment for African mothers' and that other communities were to provide services for their own ethnic groups.[70] Again when the British government increased its grant in aid to the ZMA, in the light of the increased costs associated with the opening of the Mwembeladu Maternity Home, it reiterated to the general meeting that its grant was 'given *only* in respect of free services to poor natives'.[71] Thus community parochialism – but particularly British antipathy and apprehension of Indian and Arab prosperity and local influence – undermined the ultimate effectiveness of the ZMA. The Honourable Chief Secretary of the ZMA (a British representative, but not of the medical department) level-headedly summarised the situation as follows in 1937:

All of you know how the Association started – to meet a very serious need in the town – and it would be deplorable if the public spirit and efforts made in the earlier days were to be defeated by any failure to come to some workable arrangement for carrying on the work of the Association. Naturally the communities who are chiefly concerned ask for an effective say in the affairs of the Association, but at the same time as a large annual grant of public funds is involved it is essential that the Government should also be in a position to ensure that the money is applied effectively. It is the difficulty of reconciling these two principles which has led to a good deal of trouble.[72]

Worries about excessive Indian and Arab representation in the ZMA also found their resonance in downbeat British comments about the midwifery services provided. It was felt that 'the pay of midwives who attend the non-African population of the Town is ... extremely high', not least as it was 'in excess of the maximum salary of a government European Nursing Sister, and is out of all proportion to services rendered'.[73] Zanzibar was characterised by members of the British medical administration as not having the necessary 'raw material' in terms of young women to be trained in midwifery work. As government Medical Officer Dr Leslie Webb pointed out in 1934: 'A *sine qua non* of a successful midwifery service is a staff of competent and respectable midwives.'[74] Any sort of rural maternity provision, he argued, had to provide culturally relevant midwifes, which in the rural areas of Zanzibar meant they should be 'a village Swahili'.[75] It is not that Webb was wrong in characterising the needs of rural communities thus, but rather, that the British continually emphasised the African cause. In stark contrast, the ZMA felt that it could not really invest too much effort in training African midwives, because the majority Arab and Indian women would 'object to the presence of pupil midwives at their accouchements, especially if the midwife is African'.[76]

The British, in theory at least, were much more concerned with providing rural healthcare for Africans than healthcare for the cosmopolitan (and politically active) communities of Zanzibar town, but obviously this was a selective and inconsistent claim. When the Colonial Medical Service had an opportunity to cooperate with the ZMA in its ambitions to establish a network of rural maternity health centres in 1933, the British declined to become involved because they were unable to dominate the rural expansion programme.

The British denial of their responsibility towards the Indian and Arab communities of Zanzibar in their dealings with the ZMA betrays a curious tension in colonial circles. In other realms the British actively pursued a policy of cooperation with the island's Arab elite, who were acknowledged as vital to the island's economy and political stability.

The struggles for control of the ZMA therefore highlight some of the internal dynamics of the colonial encounter which are rarely explored: namely the racial hierarchies constructed by the British towards the heterogeneous populations of the island. Of course European health was the tantamount concern, but in terms of the indigenes it was Africans, from the British perspectives, that were most deserving of their help and charity.

Conclusion

At one level this account reveals a very sorry local story of thwarted good intentions. As Colonial Medical Officer Dr Sydney Lee ruefully admitted in a private letter (a rather bitter irony, considering the trouble he has directly caused the ZMA through his allegations against it): 'I find the whole history of the Zanzibar Maternity Association, Home, Dispensary and Rural Centres most depressing reading as it is simply an account of how excellent intentions were wrecked by faction fighting.'[77] From another perspective, this case provides an appealing local example of the role played by networks of neighbourhood patronage in building and sustaining a competing organisation of healthcare, supplementing and extending historical accounts of indigenous 'resistance' to colonial medical interventions.[78]

In a broader context, however, this study shows the highly manipulative and selective way the British applied their policies of health. This in turn reveals the way colonial governance embodied elements of stagecraft – ultimately always serving a broader racial-political agenda. The Colonial Medical Service had been trying to 'facilitate the acquisition of ... control' of the ZMA since the significance of its contribution to the care of maternal health in Zanzibar Town became apparent with opening of the Mwembeladu home in 1925.[79] Clearly, to the directors of the Colonial Medical Service issues of control and dominance were more important than ideals of medical philanthropy. What is more, in justifying their withdrawal of support for the ZMA in the late 1920s and 1930s, the British used various methods to undermine its reputation. They criticised its management committee, they condemned its rural health initiatives and they discredited its midwife training programmes. Furthermore, they openly criticised the ZMA for principally supporting Indian and Arab women, seemingly oblivious to the implication that colonial medical services were principally for African populations.

Events within the ZMA's short history provide an opportunity to unravel the different British approaches towards an ethnically heterogeneous society. Although it was the majority African poor who were considered the least cultured in both British and Arab discourses, it was the Arabs and Indians who were revealed to be the most problematic within the official British stance towards the ZMA's approach to health reform. In its most simple terms this selective bias undermined Arab and Asiatic ambitions for the ZMA and suited British ambitions over its control. When the hegemony of state medicine was threatened, the British were prepared to manipulate their response so as to protect themselves from any competition.

Notes

1   Abdul Sheriff, 'The Spatial Dichotomy of Swahili Towns: The Case of Zanzibar in the Nineteenth Century', *Azania*, 67, 2002, pp. 63–81, at p. 63

2   Trading wealth was based on a prosperous dhow trade in spices and ivory (and to 1897, in slaves). See Erik Gilbert, *Dhows and the Colonial Economy in Zanzibar: 1860–1970*, Oxford, James Currey, 2004; Abdul Sheriff, *Slaves, Spices and Ivory in Zanzibar: Integration of an East African Commercial Empire into the World Economy, 1770–1873*, London, James Currey, 1987

3   Patrick Brantlinger, 'Victorians and Africans: The Genealogy of the Myth of the Dark Continent', *Critical Inquiry* 12, 1985, pp. 166–203

4   Jonathon Glassman, 'Slower than a Massacre: The Multiple Sources of Racial Thought in Colonial Africa', *American Historical Review*, 109, 2004, pp. 720–54, at p. 734

5   R. Coupland, 'Zanzibar: an Asiatic Spice Island, Kirk and Slavery, *The Times*, 5 October 1928, p. 15

6   David Livingstone, *Last Journals, 1866–88*, quoted in Andrew Balfour and Henry Harold Scott, *Health Problems of the Empire: Past, Present and Future*, London, W. Collins Sons and Co., Ltd., 1924, p. 97

7   Scott, *Health Problems of the Empire*, 1924, p. 95

8   Denise Roth Allen, *Managing Motherhood, Managing Risk: Fertility and Danger in West Central Tanzania*, Ann Arbor, University of Michigan Press, 2002; Valarie Fildes, Lara Marks and Hilary Marland (eds.), *Women and Children First: International Maternal and Infant Welfare, 1870–1945*, London, Routledge, 1992; Sarah Hodges, *Contraception, Colonialism and Commerce: Birth Control in South India, 1920–1940*, Aldershot, Ashgate, 2008; Michael Jennings, '"A Matter of Vital Importance": The Place of Medical Mission in Maternal and Child Healthcare in Tanganyika, 1919–39', in David Hardiman (ed.), *Healing Bodies, Saving Souls: Medical Missions in Asia and Africa*, Amsterdam and New York, Rodopi, pp. 227–50

9   For the neglected history of Indian doctors in East Africa see Anna Greenwood and Harshad Topiwala, *Indian Doctors in Kenya: The Forgotten Story, 1895–1940*, London, Palgrave Macmillan, 2015

10 There is a long history of generalisation about the common traits of ethnic groups. See Nicholas Hudson, 'From "Nation" to "Race": The Origin of Racial Classification in Eighteenth-Century Thought', *Eighteenth- Century Studies*, 29, 1996, pp. 247–64, at p. 249

11 'Appendix IV Fifteenth Annual Report of the Zanzibar Maternity Association for the Year Ending 31st December 1933', in Zanzibar Protectorate, *Annual Medical Report, 1933*, Zanzibar, Government Printer, 1934, pp. 77–82, at p. 77

12 Zanzibar National Archives (ZNA) AJ/29/248 Twentieth Annual Report of the Zanzibar Maternity Association for the Year Ending 31st December 1938, p. 2

13 ZNA AB/2/259 Letter from P.P. Balsara, Honorary Secretary, ZMA to Chief Secretary [no date, c. Spring, 1942]

14 Richard Hayes Crofton, *Zanzibar Affairs*, 1914–1933, London, Francis Edwards, 1953, p. 18

15 Zanzibar Protectorate, *Annual Medical Report, 1918*, Zanzibar, Government Printer, 1920. The ZMA was first mentioned in government AMRs in 1922 and thereafter short supportive statements appeared annually until 1930. Between 1923 and 1933 the annual report of the ZMA was published as an appendix to the governmental annual report. After 1933, notably less mention of the ZMA is made in the annual reports, indicating an official distancing from Association affairs and an increasing desire to see its own maternity initiatives as separate.

16 ZNA AB/2/259 Letter Dr Leslie Webb to Honorary Chief Secretary 29 July 1935. On establishment of the ZMA in 1918 both the acting British resident and the sultan were joint patrons. Hayes Crofton, *Zanzibar Affairs*, p. 15

17 Before 1928 the president was usually the highest-ranking medical official on the island, after that time, presidents included S.B.B. McElderry, of the Colonial Agricultural Service and W. Hendry, of the Colonial Education Service.

18 Zanzibar Protectorate, *Annual Medical Report, 1922*, Zanzibar, Government Printer, 1923, p. 7

19 Although it was said that fees actually averaged around 56 shillings per case when remissions and exemptions were considered. ZNA AJ/29/248 Eighteenth Annual Report of the Zanzibar Maternity Association for the Year Ending 31st December 1936

20 The Wakf Commission briefly suspended its grant between 1922 and 1925, however. ZNA HD/10/17 Sixth Annual Report of the Zanzibar Maternity Association for the Year Ending 31 December 1924. Spellings of 'wakf' varied, sometimes being 'waqf'.

21 Laura Fair, *Pastimes and Politics: Culture, Community, and Identity in Post-abolition Urban Zanzibar, 1890–1945*, Athens, OH and Oxford: Ohio University Press and James Currey, 2001, p. 123

22 ZNA AB/2/259 *Zanzibar Official Gazette*, 14 July 1928

23 ZNA AJ/29/248 Report of Meeting Held on 9 January 1937 to Discuss the Draft Articles of the Association of the Zanzibar Maternity Association, p. 2

24 ZNA AB/2/259 Letter from Leslie Webb to Honorary Chief Secretary, 29 July 1935

25 Struggles for Mwembeladu also fit in with broader struggles of the British government, via the Wakf Commission, to privatise wakf property. Fair, *Pastimes and Politics*, p. 124

26 Hayes Crofton, *Zanzibar Affairs*, p. 17

27 ZNA AB/2/259 Letter from Leslie Webb to Honorary Chief Secretary, 29 July 1935

28 ZNA AJ/25/3 Reserved Articles of the Association, 1937

29 'Appendix IV Fourteenth Annual Report of the Zanzibar Maternity Association, for the Year Ending 31st December 1932', in Zanzibar Protectorate, *Annual Medical Report, 1932*, Zanzibar, Government Printer, 1933, pp. 71–4, at p. 72

30 ZNA AB/2/259 Letter from Leslie Webb to Honorary Chief Secretary 9 October 1934

31 Zanzibar Protectorate, *Annual Medical Report, 1934*, Zanzibar, Government Printer, 1935, p. 30

32 ZNA AB/2/259 Letter from Dr Leslie Webb to Honorary Chief Secretary 19 September 1934. The final home was recommended to be closed down two years later, in 1936. ZNA AB/2/259 Memo Dr Leslie Webb to Honorary Chief Secretary 26 November 1936

33 ZNA AB/2/259 Letter from Dr Leslie Webb to Honorary Chief Secretary 19 September 1934

34 ZNA AJ/29/248 Letter from Acting Provincial Commissioner to Chief Secretary, Zanzibar, 4 May 1939

35 ZNA AB/2/259 Letter from Dr Leslie Webb to Honourable Chief Secretary [no date c. October/November 1936]

36 ZNA AB/2/259 Letter from Dr Leslie Webb to Honourable Chief Secretary, 29 July 1935

37 ZNA AJ/29/248 Report of Meeting Held on 9 January 1937 to Discuss the Draft Articles of the Association of the Zanzibar Maternity Association, p. 2

38   ZNA AJ/25/3 Reserved Articles of the Association, 1937
39   Zanzibar Protectorate, *Annual Medical Report, 1937*, Zanzibar, Government Printer, 1938, p. 37
40   ZNA AB/2/259 Letter Dr Lee to Chief Secretary, 12 June 1939
41   ZNA AJ/29/248 Letter from Acting Provincial Commissioner to Honourable Chief Secretary, 17 June 1939
42   ZNA AJ/29/248 Letter from Acting Provincial Commissioner to Honourable Chief Secretary, 17 June 1939
43   ZNA AJ/29/248 Letter from Miss B.J. Locket to Mr J. O'Brien, President, ZMA, 9 April 1943
44   ZNA AJ/29/248 Minute Dr J.C. Earl to Honorary Chief Secretary, 5 February 1944. See also ZNA AJ/29/248 Zanzibar Maternity Association, Minutes of the Meeting of the Executive Committee, 9 June 1947
45   Zanzibar Protectorate, *Annual Medical Report, 1928*, Zanzibar, Government Printer, 1929, p. 38
46   Zanzibar Protectorate, *Annual Medical Report, 1922*, p. 4
47   Balfour and Scott, *Health Problems of the Empire*, pp. 323–32
48   Margaret Jones, *Health Policy in Britain's Model Colony: Ceylon (1900–1948)*, New Delhi, Orient Longman, 2004. Although Anna Davin has argued that British interest in maternal and child health in Britain's imperial possessions began around 1900. Anna Davin, 'Imperialism and Motherhood', in Frederick Cooper and Ann Laura Stoler (eds.), *Tensions of Empire: Colonial Cultures in a Bourgeois World*, Berkeley, University of California Press, 1997, pp. 87–151, esp. pp. 93–7
49   Zanzibar Protectorate, *Annual Medical Report, 1924*, Zanzibar, Government Printer, 1925, p. 42–3; see also, Zanzibar Protectorate, *Annual Medical Report, 1925*, Zanzibar, Government Printer, 1926, p. 31
50   ZNA AJ/27/705 Personnel File: Dr Violet Ruth Sharp. Sharp retired when she married in 1942, and was succeeded in 1943 by Dr Elizabeth Harrison. See ZNA AJ/27/596 Personnel File: Dr Elizabeth Nora Harrison
51   Dr Muriel Robertson. See Anna Crozier, *Practising Colonial Medicine: the Colonial Medical Service in British East Africa*, London, I.B. Tauris, 2007, p. 98. A discussion is also included here of WMOs in Kenya, Uganda and Tanzania more broadly. For the development of maternal health services in Nigeria see Deanne van Tol, 'Mothers, Babies, and the Colonial State: The Introduction of Maternal and Infant Welfare Services in Nigeria, 1925–1945', *Spontaneous Generations*, 1, 2007, pp. 110–31
52   ZNA AB/2/259 Letter from Dr Leslie Webb to Honorary Chief Secretary, 23 October 1934
53   ZNA AB/2/259 Letter from Dr J. Lee to Chief Secretary, ZMA, 11 July 1939
54   Warwick Anderson, 'Excremental Colonialism: Public Health and the Poetics of Pollution', *Critical Enquiry*, 21, 1995, pp. 640–69; Warwick Anderson, *Colonial Pathologies: American Tropical Medicine, Race and Hygiene in the Philippines*, Durham, NC, Duke University Press, 2006; Anna Crozier, 'Sensationalising Africa: British Medical Impressions of Sub-Saharan Africa 1890–1939', *Journal of Imperial and Commonwealth History*, 35, 2007, pp. 393–415; Megan Vaughan, *Curing Their Ills: Colonial Power and African Illness*, Cambridge, Polity Press, 1991. This list is far from exhaustive.
55   'Zanzibar Maternity Association', *Zanzibar Official Gazette* (Supplement), 14 July 1926
56   Zanzibar Protectorate, *Annual Medical Report, 1927*, Zanzibar, Government Printer, 1928, p. 7
57   Zanzibar Protectorate, *Annual Medical Report, 1930*, Zanzibar, Government Printer, 1931, p. 5
58   Hayes Crofton, *Zanzibar Affairs*, p. 15
59   Other examples of British selective policy making towards the different categories of colonial subjects on Zanzibar can be found in Geoffrey Ross Owens, 'Exploring the Articulation of Governmentality and Sovereignty: The Chwaka Road and the Bombardment of Zanzibar', *Journal of Colonialism and Colonial History*, 8, 2007,

pp. 1–55; Friedhelm Hartwig, 'The Segmentation of the Indian Ocean Region. Arabs and the Implementation of Immigration Regulations in Zanzibar and British East Africa', in Jan-Georg Deutsch and Brigitte Reinwald (eds.), *Space on the Move. Transformations of the Indian Ocean Seascape in the Nineteenth and Twentieth Century*, Berlin, Klaus Schwarz Verlag, 2002, pp. 21–35

60   Jonathon Glassman, 'Sorting out the Tribes: The Creation of Racial Identities in Colonial Zanzibar's Newspaper Wars', *Journal of African History*, 41, 2000, pp. 395–428

61   ZNA AJ/29/248 Letter from Acting Provincial Commissioner to Chief Secretary, Zanzibar, 4 May 1939

62   Zanzibar Protectorate, *Annual Medical Report, 1922*, p. 7; ZNA AJ/29/248 Nineteenth Annual Report of the Zanzibar Maternity Association for the Year Ending 31 December 1937, pp. 1–2

63   E.g. in 1936 the Hindu Mandal ceased its contribution to the ZMA because it wanted its money to support only members of the Hindu community, except those of the Bhattia sect – a distinction which proved almost impossible to police. ZNA AJ/29/248 Eighteenth Annual Report of the Zanzibar Maternity Association for the Year Ending 31st December 1936

64   ZNA AJ/29/248 Nineteenth Annual Report of the Zanzibar Maternity Association for the Year Ending 31st December 1937, pp. 1–2

65   ZNA AJ/29/248 Zanzibar Maternity Association Jan 1937–June 1947, Letter from Provincial Commissioner to Chief Secretary, 21 October 1942. This should also be seen as part of a growing nationalist debate on the Arab elites on Zanzibar (Arab Association founded 1911). Even though this group did not directly speak in explicitly racial terms, it did mobilise a polemic of ethnic exclusionism that sought to favour urban Arabs over Africans of mainland origin. Glassman, 'Slower than a Massacre', p. 236

66   My emphasis: Zanzibar Protectorate, *Annual Medical Report, 1921*, Zanzibar, Government Printer, 1922, pp. 28–9

67   Zanzibar Protectorate, *Annual Medical Report, 1921*, p. 33

68   Zanzibar Protectorate, *Annual Medical Report, 1923*, Zanzibar, Government Printer, 1924, p. 80

69   ZNA AJ/29/248 Zanzibar Maternity Association Jan 1937–June 1947, Letter from Provincial Commissioner to Chief Secretary, 21 October 1942

70   ZNA AB/2/259 Letter from Dr Leslie Webb to Honorary Chief Secretary, 29 July 1935

71   ZNA AB/2/259 Letter from Dr Leslie Webb to Honorary Chief Secretary, 29 July 1935, my emphasis.

72   ZNA AJ/29/248 Report of Meeting Held on 9th January 1937 to Discuss the Draft of Articles of the Association of the Zanzibar Maternity Association, pp. 1–2

73   ZNA AB/2/259 Letter from Dr Leslie Webb to Honorary Chief Secretary, 19 September 1934

74   ZNA AB/2/259 Letter from Dr Leslie Webb to Honorary Chief Secretary, 23 October 1934

75   ZNA AB/2/259 Letter from Dr Leslie Webb to Honorary Chief Secretary, 23 October 1934

76   ZNA AJ/12/35 Memo from Dr W.M. Lewis to SMO, 15 July 1942

77   ZNA AB/2/259 Letter from Dr S.W. Lee to Honorary Chief Secretary, 28 April 1939

78   David Arnold, *Colonizing the Body: State Medicine and Epidemic Disease in Nineteenth-Century India*, Berkeley, University of California Press, 1993

79   ZNA AB/2/259 Letter from Dr Leslie Webb to Honorary Chief Secretary, 7 July 1934

CHAPTER SIX

Elder Dempster and the transport of lunatics in British West Africa

Matthew M. Heaton

In 1954 a Nigerian man named L.S. arrived in the United Kingdom to study carpentry at the L.C.C. School of Building in Brixton.[1] Within eight months of his arrival in the UK, L.S. suffered a mental breakdown. In April 1955 he was admitted to the Warlingham Park Hospital, having developed a 'strong persecution mania'.[2] Hospital attendants described him as 'extremely depressed, agitated and unsure of his surrounding'. He claimed he was about to die and that he heard voices calling his name in his native language.[3] With auditory hallucinations ongoing in a patient saddled with what his doctor termed 'an inadequate and dependent personality', his British doctors determined that it was 'unwise to encourage his continued stay in this country' and recommended that he return to Nigeria for further care.[4] On 23 February 1956, L.S. sailed on the Elder Dempster ship *Apapa*, arriving in Lagos some twenty-one days later, repatriated under paid escort at the expense of the government of the United Kingdom.

L.S.'s repatriation was not unique. Over the course of the British colonial era in Nigeria, which lasted from roughly 1900 to 1960, hundreds of immigrant Nigerians succumbed to mental disorders while living outside of Nigeria. Many dozens were repatriated as a result, supposedly in their own best interests to optimise their recovery. Repatriation of those deemed mentally ill was, however, a complicated process involving a variety of medical, governmental and corporate authorities, not least of which was the shipping firm of Elder Dempster & Company, which held a virtual monopoly over the carrying trade between the UK and its West African colonies for more or less the entirety of Nigeria's colonial history. This chapter examines the relationship between Elder Dempster and the medical and governmental authorities within the British Empire. I argue here that this relationship represents an example of the importance of public-private cooperation in the maintenance of the medical geography of Empire, even as it reveals significant tensions underlying such cooperation.

Histories of psychiatry in colonial settings remain significantly state centred.[5] However, historical and anthropological studies of health and illness in Africa more broadly have established quite definitively that the state by no means controlled the ways that knowledge about health and illness was created and interpolated in colonial and post-colonial environments. [6] Indeed, the important and sometimes influential role of non-state actors in the development of psychiatric science has been increasingly recognised in more contemporary contexts, as psycho-pharmaceutical companies exert influence on both medical and state authorities, shaping the very understanding of the diseases that their products treat and blurring the line between patient and market.[7] However, the pharmaceutical industry's motivation for inserting itself into debates about mental health and illness is in many ways much more direct and its impact much more obvious than that of Elder Dempster. This chapter thus seeks to look 'beyond the state' by expanding upon the understanding of the indirect role that capitalist enterprises have played in reinforcing imperialist notions about the relationship between citizenship, psychopathology and cultural geography in the British Empire.

The first section of the chapter makes the case that Elder Dempster's role in transporting mentally ill Nigerians allowed for the implementation of colonial psychiatric theories about the nature of mental illness in Africans in ways that would have otherwise been unfeasible. As such, Elder Dempster was engaged in a medical procedure as much as in a commercial shipping transaction. Repatriation was a vector of therapy similar to the syringe used in an injection or the capsule holding the active ingredients of a pharmaceutical concoction. Transporting mentally ill Nigerians was not just a political or economic expediency. In the context of colonial psychiatric theories that emphasised the psychological threats of cross-cultural exchange, returning mentally ill migrants to the geographical spaces where they 'belonged' was itself a means to a therapeutic end. Elder Dempster was therefore a role player in the medical infrastructure of the British Empire, just as it was in the facilitation of administrative and commercial networks.

The second section of the chapter moves from discussing the cohesive role of Elder Dempster as a medical collaborator to examine the tensions that arose from utilising a public-private relationship for such purposes. Organising repatriations of mentally ill immigrants revealed underlying tensions between the practice of colonial medicine (or, more accurately, the practice of medicine on colonial subjects), the legal rights of British colonial subjects and the corporate liabilities of privately held businesses like Elder Dempster. Despite the fact that Elder Dempster was performing this medical procedure (repatriation) on behalf of the government, it was not itself a government agency and, as such, never enjoyed the coercive powers of the state. As we will see, legally speaking, passengers on Elder Dempster lines could not be certified mental patients, despite the fact that they were being transported for psychiatric purposes. This made the prospect of transporting unstable individuals somewhat unappetising for the company. However, Elder Dempster also desired to maintain good relations with the British government and to continue to enjoy a privileged position as a monopoly over public shipping to and from West Africa. This sometimes required engaging in risky endeavours that the company would otherwise eschew based on strictly commercial grounds. Negotiations over the appropriate procedures for carrying out repatriations therefore became tense and their results somewhat nebulous from a policy standpoint, but they nevertheless usually resulted in the repatriation of the patient in question. Thus, in more than one way Elder Dempster became a 'go-between' for the British Empire. The company quite literally linked the physical spaces of the UK, Nigeria and other West African colonies, while it also figuratively inhabited the space between the will of government and medical authorities, on the one hand and the legal rights of their passenger-patients, on the other.

Elder Dempster, Nigerian 'lunatics' and the medical geography of Empire

This section examines the ways in which Elder Dempster's involvement in the repatriation of mentally ill Nigerians were seen as part of a medical procedure designed specifically to address the psychological turmoil of the patient-passengers to whom it was prescribed and which medical authorities were ill-equipped to carry out on their own. In so doing, it addresses the construction of a medical geography of Empire that defined colonial subjects as psychologically suited to particular spaces and threatened by the crossing of cultural boundaries. Colonial medical departments across British-controlled Africa had played an extremely important role in developing this medical geography. They had established asylums throughout British Africa for the confinement of particularly violent and dangerous 'insane' colonial subjects and in so doing had created the space within which colonial ethnopsychiatrists developed theories about the nature of the 'African mind' that defined the African in general racial terms as mentally inferior to the European and therefore psychologically threatened by European 'civilisation'. These theories, developed within the structures and institutions of colonial medical departments and, frequently, through the research and pronouncements of colonial medical officials (among others), filtered out from the colonies to affect the way medical and governmental officials in the United Kingdom thought about the causes of mental illness in immigrant Nigerians. However, it was through negotiations between the Colonial Office and Elder Dempster that repatriations were mostly arranged, with the colonial medical department in Nigeria playing only a minor role in confirming or denying accommodation for the patient on his return. But through these negotiations Elder Dempster became integral in the realisation of a medical process that colonial medical departments could not have enforced on their own: that of removing immigrant Nigerians from a society that was presumed to be psychologically damaging and returning them to cultural surroundings – and possibly the care of colonial medical authorities – in the places where they 'belonged'.

Migration was a cornerstone of European empires in Africa in the nineteenth and twentieth centuries. Over the course of time African subjects of European empires migrated within colonies from rural areas to urban areas, from areas with depressed economies to places where jobs were available, and from places far removed from the centres of power, wealth and education to places of greater opportunity.[8] Nigerians were no exception to this rule. In the early twentieth century, most migration of Nigerians took place within Nigeria and to neighbouring colonies in West Africa. Some, however, travelled to Great Britain, the United States or other Western countries as students, soldiers, or wage labourers in the shipping industry. Still others travelled eastwards, fulfilling their Muslim duty of pilgrimage to Mecca.

It is difficult to know at what rates Nigerian immigrants fell victim to mental illnesses severe enough to warrant the attention of medical authorities, and certainly the medical and governmental gaze varied in emphasis across space and time. Nevertheless, evidence exists that Nigerians whom local authorities deemed to have lost control of their mental faculties were present in all of these regions of the world.[9] As early as 1916, British colonial authorities in the Gold Coast (Ghana) sought unsuccessfully to repatriate sixteen Nigerians resident in the mental asylum in Accra.[10] In 1927, France unsuccessfully sought to repatriate a mentally ill African named M.Q., supposedly of Nigerian origin, who had suffered a brain injury as a soldier in the First World War and somehow found his way to Paris, where he was living in conditions of 'starvation and exposure'.[11] But by far the most prevalent source of documented requests for repatriation of Nigerian mental cases came from the UK, and came in the post-Second World War period as increasing numbers of Nigerians travelled to the UK for work and higher education.[12] Although repatriation requests from before 1945 show scant documentation and were rarely successful, repatriations from the UK in the post-war era were commonly executed, and the repatriated mental patients almost always travelled home on an Elder Dempster ship.

Elder Dempster's indispensable role in linking the UK and its West African colonies in terms of commerce, communications and passenger traffic stems from the twinned growth of steam shipping and the extension of the British Empire into West Africa in the second half of the nineteenth century. The first major British shipping mogul in West Africa was Macgregor Laird, who famously started the African Steamship Company in 1852, just one year after the British had officially annexed Lagos. Laird's company was primarily interested in the palm-oil trade in the Niger river area, but also called at a variety of other West African ports and in the 1850s became the official mail carrier between the UK and West Africa. In 1868, two former employees of Laird's Liverpool agents, Alexander Elder and John Dempster, founded a competing firm, named the British and African Steam Navigation Company. A third employee of the African Steamship Company, Alfred Jones, began his own line in 1878, and began chartering goods to West Africa in 1879. Jones's early success resulted in Elder and Dempster bringing him on as a partner, forming Elder Dempster & Co. as agents of the British and African Steam Navigation Company. Jones became the senior partner and chairman of Elder Dempster in 1884 and worked to build Elder Dempster into the pre-eminent shipping firm for the British West Africa trade. Through the establishment of partnerships, stock purchases, and a shipping conference with its competitors, Elder Dempster established an almost complete monopoly over the carrying trade between the UK and West Africa by the turn of the twentieth century.[13]

This monopoly included the carriage of passengers. Olukoju has noted that, while official passenger data are hard to come by, it is likely that most passenger traffic was directly related to colonial governance, particularly the movement of colonial officials and their families booked at government expense. By the 1920s, with an increase in competition from foreign shippers in the wake of the First World War, the British government instituted a policy requiring all government bookings for passengers to and from West Africa be made through the British-owned Elder Dempster line.[14] Although many officials balked at this policy because Elder Dempster did not always provide the cheapest, fastest or most comfortable passenger service, the policy remained in place through the 1950s. Therefore, when the British government wanted to repatriate Nigerian mental patients, it was bound to do

[108]

so through Elder Dempster as a first resort, and Elder Dempster had every motivation to work with the government to illustrate that this privilege was deserved.

But why ask Elder Dempster to carry out the repatriation of Nigerian mental patients? Nigerians were British subjects, after all, and had full right of residency in the UK. They were legally entitled to live, work and receive medical care indefinitely in British-controlled territories and could not be compelled to return to their native homes against their will, even if they were certified mental patients. One might assume that the first and most obvious option was to care for them in hospital in the UK, providing treatment and accommodation until such point as they were capable of looking after themselves. Indeed, the spirit of both British and British West African law throughout the colonial period held that 'wherever people become lunatics, there they remain'.[15] Even after repatriation of Nigerian mental patients became commonplace from the UK in the 1950s, some colonial officials wondered what was the reasoning behind the procedure. Nigerian medical infrastructure certainly could not rival that of the 'imperial motherland'. Psychiatric facilities in Nigeria were particularly unpleasant, characterised as overcrowded, understaffed and offering nothing in the way of therapeutic care.[16] The disparity was stark enough that one Nigerian official queried,

> I presume there must be full legal sanction for banishing these unfortunate people from Britain? Their fate on returning here must in most cases be pitiable ... if they do not return home as useless and despised members of their own communities they have mostly, as the only alternative, to be confined in crowded and deplorable sections of prisons reserved for those in such a plight.[17]

That repatriation of British subjects to their lands of origin was a reasonable way to handle cases of psychological disorder was certainly neither a legal nor a medical inevitability.

The motivations for repatriating Nigerians who developed mental illnesses in the UK were based to a certain extent on financial concerns. British officials often saw the expenses incurred in their daily maintenance of non-native British subjects in their local hospitals and asylums as an undue burden on government resources. Financial considerations, however, were not sufficient to justify the relocation of a certified mental patient. Based on British and British West African law, mental patients could not be moved if the primary motivation was government convenience. British subjects could be repatriated only if medical authorities agreed that such repatriation would likely result in an improvement in the patient's material circumstances or medical condition. Luckily for government officials who had a vested financial interest in repatriating Nigerian mental patients, in many cases medical authorities were, indeed, of the opinion that repatriation should improve the mental health of unstable Nigerians.

The medical justification for repatriating Nigerian mental patients was deeply rooted in ideological perspectives on the relationship between race, culture and human psychology that developed in the context of a European imperialism that sought to explain the power dynamics of Empire in scientific terms.[18] The literature on race and colonialism is abundant, and beyond the scope of this chapter, other than to say that the cultural politics upon which the British Empire were based in the first half of the twentieth century overwhelmingly cast the European coloniser as the arbiter of justice, decency, intelligence, rationality and 'civilisation', in diametric contrast to black Africans' presumed injustice, indecency, unintelligence, irrationality and overall primitivity. While innate biological differences were strongly purported to account for the perceived disparity between white and black races early in the twentieth century, particularly through the findings of eugenicists like H.L. Gordon, H.W. Vint and their cohort in the East African school, by the 1930s, anthropologists and social scientists had begun to explain the difference between the races largely in cultural terms.

Psychology and psychiatry had an important role to play in defining the differences between social and cultural systems and, ultimately, the presumed effects of culture on the psychological and intellectual processes of individuals.[19] Pseudo-scientific studies created the impression that the black and white races were, if not innately different, at least very far apart in terms of cultural evolution. Such a presumption allowed for an explanation of European will to power in African environments in terms other than exploitation and extraordinary violence. However, it also created a context in which European scientists, anthropologists and, ultimately, colonial officials became preoccupied with the presumed consequences of the 'clash of cultures' that emerged when Europeans and Africans came into contact. If the intellectual and cultural nature of the European was inclined towards justice, order and progress, then this psychological predisposition would be significantly frustrated and or/degraded by living in the African's diametrically opposite socio-cultural milieu. The trope of 'going native' so famously embodied by Joseph Conrad's Kurtz in *Heart of Darkness* was representative of real concerns amongst Europeans about the psychological consequences of imperial domination. In fact, British West African colonial governments had developed *de facto* policies for the repatriation of Europeans who developed mental illnesses in Africa long before

[110]

they ever contemplated having to repatriate Africans from Europe.[20] For example, British and American medical thought frequently identified geographic locale as contributory to the causes of a nervous condition in whites living in tropical environments known as 'tropical neurasthenia'. Repatriation of white neurasthenics became a common political, social and medical remedy to the problems posed by a mental illness presumably caused by exposure to alien environments.[21]

If crossing these racial-cum-cultural boundaries was a psychological threat to Europeans, the consequences were heightened for Africans. European colonialism in Africa brought significant upheavals of political, economic and cultural traditions of African societies. For European ethnopsychiatrists, such upheaval was a good thing in the long term, as it would bring Africans closer to the level of 'civilisation' that Europeans enjoyed. However, it posed serious short-term psychological consequences for Africans ill equipped to handle the transition from a presumably unchanging, 'traditional' existence to a highly dynamic 'modern' world. Although there were a few detractors, psychological studies of Africans before the 1960s tended to support the notion that, in general, adult African intelligence was inferior to that of the adult European. Inferior intelligence was deemed to be both a cause and a consequence of cultures that failed to produce productive, introspective individuals. Unlike in European cultures, which valued individuality, ambition and self-awareness, ethnopsychiatrists argued that African cultures emphasised conformity, communalism and the sublimation of the individual to the community and the supernatural. For acclaimed ethnopsychiatrists like J.C. Carothers, the communally oriented, extroverted, unambitious, superstitious, unintelligent African lacking introspective insight and living only in the present and without a care for the future became the default definition of the 'normal' African.[22]

Mental illnesses in Africans were characterised by deviation from this norm. As Megan Vaughan has noted, the 'mad African' was frequently constructed as the 'colonial subject who was insufficiently "Other" – who spoke of being rich, of hearing voices through radio sets, of being powerful, who imitated the white man in dress and behaviour'.[23] In other words, Africans who deviated from their 'traditional' norms and blurred the arbitrary cultural boundaries between white European and black African were considered the most psychologically vulnerable segment of African populations. Ethnopsychiatrists dubbed the adoption of European norms by Africans 'deculturation' or 'detribalisation', and considered it amongst the biggest threats to African mental health by the 1950s.

Such conditions were seen to be an encroaching threat in African spaces as a result of colonisation. However, when an African travelled away from his native home, particularly to Europe, the heart of modern civilisation, the psychological stakes were obviously raised further. By the 1950s, psychiatrists and social scientists were beginning to show serious concern over the perceived high levels of mental breakdown amongst West Africans in the UK. Both Margaret Field, an anthropologist working in Gold Coast, and Raymond Prince, a psychiatrist working in Nigeria in the late 1950s, expressed concern over the recognisable preponderance of psychiatric disturbance amongst West Africans who travelled to the UK for higher education.[24] Studies conducted in the UK on psychiatric morbidity in student populations seemed to uphold the idea that Nigerian students were particularly vulnerable to mental breakdown while abroad. For example, in a 1960 study of mental health in overseas students at Leeds University R.J. Still found that Nigerian students had a more than double rate of 'psychological reactions' – ranging from the 'severe' to the 'trivial' – than native British students.[25] In a later study, Cecil B. Kidd, of the Department of Psychiatric Medicine at Edinburgh University, saw similar results, with conspicuously high rates of mental breakdown amongst Nigerian students.[26]

Regardless of the purported 'cause' of the mental breakdown, medical authorities frequently articulated that their Nigerian patients were incapable of recovering in an alien cultural environment like that of the UK and, frequently, that returning to more familiar cultural surroundings would be psychologically beneficial. Repatriation was, then, not just a means for the British government to save taxpayer money, *it was constructed as a medical intervention in its own right.* Take, for example, the case of M.O., a nineteen-year-old Nigerian admitted to Saxondale Hospital in Nottingham with schizophrenia who applied for repatriation in 1950. The hospital staff supported the repatriation on the grounds that 'the boy is unlikely to make a full recovery until he gets home'.[27] Similarly, G.N., a twenty-six-year-old patient in Bristol Mental Hospital diagnosed with 'reactive depression with gross hysterical phenomena', applied for repatriation in 1952 and was supported in this decision by psychiatric authorities who considered repatriation 'essential to complete recovery'.[28] The doctor of P.A., a Nigerian 'said to be suffering from serious mental disability' in 1956 declared that 'in view of his mental condition, he would best be treated in his own country'.[29] The exact same wording was used to support the repatriation of N.U., who suffered from 'schizophrenia of an intense and paranoid type'. The consultant psychiatrist at Long Grove Hospital in Surrey informed the Colonial Office in 1958 that 'the sooner he can be repatriated the better'.[30] All of these patients were repatriated on Elder Dempster ships.

[112]

In carrying out the repatriation of Nigerian mental patients, Elder Dempster was simultaneously engaged in a medical intervention and a reinforcement of the medical geography of the British Empire that both defined particular bounded spaces as natural cultural milieus for colonial subjects of different races and at the same time articulated psychological threats for individuals who crossed those boundaries. Clearly in these cases, and the many more not described in this chapter, the repatriation of West Africans was not just an exercise of their rights as British subjects, or of their desires as alienated individuals, but also an integral part of the treatment of their mental disorder. It should also be noted that the diagnoses in the cases mentioned above were diverse, yet in all of them, repatriation was considered to be a necessary therapeutic intervention, an intervention more powerful than anything that could be provided under current circumstances in a 'modern', but nonetheless alien country. Elder Dempster played the role of helping Nigerian mental patients to at least partially 'un-cross' some of the racial and cultural boundaries that had supposedly contributed so greatly to their psychological disturbance, thereby presumably simultaneously strengthening the social health of the Empire and the health of individual patients.

Repatriating mental patients and the tensions of Empire

Elder Dempster's role in repatriating Nigerian mental patients is an illustration of the ways that business entities could be important participants in the reinforcement of the ideological underpinnings of the British Empire. Additionally, this trend should be seen as revealing of some of the anxieties of maintaining imperial order, particularly if one examines the tensions that clearly existed between Elder Dempster and the government during cases of repatriation. While desire to maintain a racially segregated social order may have implicitly motivated recommendations for repatriations, the logistics of carrying out these repatriations were not so simple. Transporting mentally ill Nigerians from the UK to their native homes proved to be a relatively complicated process that required balancing the medical needs and legal rights of the Nigerian patient with the financial constraints of government and the liability concerns of Elder Dempster, the central question being who, ultimately, was the responsible party carrying out the repatriation: the individual patient, the British government, the medical authority recommending the repatriation or Elder Dempster, on whose property the patient resided during the voyage home? On top of the difficulties posed by this question, the answer had to be agreeable to all parties and make more sense than simply not repatriating the patient at all.

[113]

This section examines these tensions, illustrating the ways that Elder Dempster's position as a private enterprise sometimes conflicted with the interests of its primary client, the British imperial government. Even within these tensions, however, we must recognise that neither Elder Dempster nor the Colonial Office particularly questioned the underlying notion that repatriation was good for mentally ill colonial subjects. They were mostly concerned with the legal contradictions of trying to give Elder Dempster – a private shipping company – the necessary coercive powers of medical and governmental authorities in order to carry out a procedure that those authorities had ordered and which Elder Dempster had agreed to execute, but for which no party wanted to take responsibility.

As mentioned above, British law did not allow for the forcible removal of any certified mental patient, regardless of race, culture or nationality, from one place within the Empire to another. In order to repatriate a non-native mental patient, the patient had first to be decertified, legally restoring all the rights and responsibilities of a normal, healthy individual. Patients then had to undergo travel to their homelands, where their psychological state could be re-evaluated on arrival. However, even after decertification from the mental hospital, no British citizen or colonial subject could be forced to return home. Consent to repatriation was a sine qua non for their removal. In most of the Nigerian cases for whom I have records, this was of little relevance, as the patient was usually keen to return home, particularly if it might mean release from a mental hospital in the UK. However, some were reluctant, even outright refusing repatriation when it was suggested to them.[31] In these cases, the possibility of repatriation was a non-starter. So it is indeed possible to make the case that individual Nigerians themselves were responsible for their own repatriations, as their consent was necessary in order for it to happen at all.

Elder Dempster, however, was not satisfied to allow mental patients returning home to travel entirely on their own recognisance. Although Elder Dempster had been repatriating mental patients from the UK and in between British West African territories since the early twentieth century, there does not seem to have been a particular policy in place for such repatriations until after the Second World War. Several bad experiences had convinced the shipping firm that the patients being repatriated on their ships were frequently far more unstable than medical or governmental authorities knew or were willing to divulge. For example, in 1945 Elder Dempster transported a man named L.L. from Accra to Lagos. L.L. had recently been decertified and discharged from the Accra Mental Hospital for the purpose of repatriating him to Nigeria. It was presumed that L.L. was fit to travel, but he made a ruckus on the voyage, causing Nigerian officials to note when he arrived that 'his behaviour en route to Lagos suggests ... that he is still liable to fits and is of a violent nature'.[32] Later, in 1950, Elder Dempster noted that 'two recent deaths' of mental patients en route from the UK to their homes in West Africa had illustrated to the company the need to have much more detailed medical histories of the mentally ill passengers it agreed to carry.[33]

Such outcomes should not necessarily be surprising. Indeed, for many of the cases mentioned above, the repatriation was implemented not as the happy ending to a medical crisis overcome but, rather, as a medical intervention in its own right, implemented in the belief that it would help to improve the health of patients who were clearly still suffering. Elder Dempster was quite aware that many of the patients suggested for repatriation remained unstable and were being decertified only for the legal purpose of putting them on a boat home, not because they were capable of looking after themselves. Carrying such passengers put Elder Dempster at some significant liability. Violent or uncontrollable passengers posed potential threats to the security of the crew and other passengers on the vessel, which reflected poorly on Elder Dempster. At the same time, Elder Dempster took on significant responsibility for the welfare of the patient during the voyage. And taking passengers with known behavioural issues without having a reasonable policy for their neutralisation on board only put the company at greater legal risk, should that patient cause any harm to person or property. Despite the legal responsibility placed on the patient for the decision to return home, Elder Dempster carried significant responsibility for making sure that the voyage went as smoothly as possible.

In order to address what it considered to be the 'somewhat unsatisfactory' experience of repatriating mental patients, Elder Dempster approached the Colonial Office in 1950 about developing a procedure that would simultaneously protect 'abnormal passengers', other voyagers on the vessel and the company itself from liability if and when things went badly.[34] In a despatch from the Colonial Office to the Crown Agents of British West Africa, the Colonial Office made it clear that Elder Dempster was 'agreeable to carry uncertified patients', and that 'normally no difficulties need arise with such bookings'. However, the company demanded that certain protocol be observed. First, suitable accommodation for the patient had to be available. Second, the person or authority making arrangements for the repatriation of the patient had to supply a case history of the patient to the ship's surgeon and make arrangements for six passengers to act as attendants for the patient at the remuneration rate of £1 a day each.[35] Finally, and most problematically, Elder Dempster was adamant that any medical directives suggested by the medical superintendent of the company for the treatment of the patient must 'be accepted on behalf of the patient' by a responsible third party.[36]

The rationale behind Elder Dempster's demands was somewhat complex. On the one hand, Elder Dempster wanted to be informed of the case history of every patient and to have consultation with the doctor previously in charge of the case in order that the company's medical superintendent might have the necessary information to make proper decisions regarding the care, treatment and accommodation of the patient during the voyage. However, on the other hand, the demand that the decisions of the medical superintendent were to be accepted on behalf of the patient suggested that the company wanted to transfer responsibility for the decisions that its employees made regarding the treatment of mentally ill patients. Simultaneously, the demand that the person or authority making arrangements for the patient also make arrangements for six attendants further guaranteed that Elder Dempster could not be held responsible for any action taken towards the patient by the very attendants that the company had demanded be there in the first place. In other words, Elder Dempster was trying to have its cake and eat it too.

Elder Dempster believed these requests to be perfectly reasonable in light of what the government was requesting of the company, i.e. the transport of unstable individuals who it knew needed serious medical attention and who could pose significant risk to other passengers and the company's reputation and assets. However, from the perspective of some British officials, some of these requests were fantastical. Legally speaking, once the patient was decertified and discharged from the mental hospital in the UK, no 'responsible party' could consent to medical directives issued by Elder Dempster on his or her behalf. The Minister of Health made clear that in such cases 'there would be no objection to a case history and a certificate being furnished', but scoffed that 'the Minister could not agree to ... being asked to make arrangements for the passage which would involve his accepting responsibility for any untoward incident which might arise on the ship'.[37] From the Colonial Office's perspective, there were 'grave doubts whether a patient could be lawfully compelled to undertake a voyage or constrained to comply with the conditions prescribed by the Medical Superintendent of the Company without his consent'.[38] The point was moot anyway, from the Colonial Office's perspective, since even if a third party took responsibility for the recommendations of the company's medical superintendent, if the patient decided to sue Elder Dempster for mistreatment 'the Company will not thereby be relieved of responsibility', because no third party had the legal authority to consent to the forced medical treatment of an individual who at the time of the voyage was not a certified mental patient.[39]

The Colonial Office ultimately considered that in most cases the authority of the ship's captain under common law would afford a 'legal justification' for the use of restraint, although not necessarily in all cases. Since no third party could provide such protection, the Colonial Office suggested that 'where it is possible ... the patient himself, or if he is under age, his parent or guardian, should be asked to give a written consent to the proposed conditions before the voyage begins'.[40] Recognising the irony of this, Elder Dempster queried the Colonial Office, 'to whom is it proposed a patient himself should give a written consent? If to an acceptable person or authority making arrangements for the voyage who in turn would instruct us in writing all well and good but we are afraid we would decline to accept any undertaking signed by a mental case, which to our mind would have no legal value.'[41] Such a statement is a clear indication from Elder Dempster that the company did not consider these patients to be worthy or even necessarily capable of personal sovereignty.

The legal peculiarities put both the Colonial Office and the company between a rock and a hard place. While it was recognised that the individuals involved in these repatriation cases were frequently not capable of making decisions for themselves, legally no one else could take responsibility for them. The Colonial Office finally relented, informing the Crown Agents that 'whether or not the patient gives such a consent, a member of his family should be asked to give his concurrence' to the company's prescribed directives. Barring a family member, 'either the person or authority making arrangements for the voyage, or the medical authority in whose charge the patient has been, must assent to the prescribed conditions on his own responsibility'.[42] In response to the legal absurdity of such an approach, the government of Nigeria pointed out the futility of the situation, declaring that 'it is not clear what advantage the Company expects to obtain', as 'the consent suggested can be of no legal avail to the Company in respect of any liability which they may incur'.[43] At best, the Nigerian government argued, such consent could be used to delude the patient, and possibly his or her family, that any actions taken were legal and that the company bore no responsibility for any outcomes resulting from their imposition. Regardless, the Nigerian government acquiesced, stating that 'if, however, such a covenant will make the Company feel easier in accepting a patient as a passenger, this Government sees no further objection to its being obtained from them'.[44] The Colonial Office also recognised the legal futility of such an arrangement for Elder Dempster's purposes. In the first draft of its despatch to the Crown Agents on the subject, the Colonial Office had urged the Crown Agents to go along with it on the grounds that it was 'unlikely that further discussions would secure terms in any way more satisfactory or precise' and that ultimately it was 'satisfactory to have received a recorded assurance from the Company of its readiness to accept bookings for mental patients'.[45] This rationale, however, was edited out of the final draft.

The procedures outlined by Elder Dempster became official policy from 1950 onward, although particulars of each case were determined on an *ad hoc* basis. Over the course of the 1950s, literally dozens of Nigerians were repatriated using these procedures. So many mental patients were being repatriated that by 1955 a colonial official in Nigeria declared that 'nearly every mail boat brings one such person'.[46] Most repatriation cases seem to have gone quite smoothly, at least from the records left behind, although problems did still arise. Nevertheless, it is important to note that the policies put in place accomplished more than securing reasonable accommodation for patients and other passengers. Although the demands made by Elder Dempster to defray responsibility for mistreatment of repatriated mental patients did not in and of themselves provide legal absolution, the heightened levels of observation and longer paper trail resulting from the institution of this policy did tend to work in Elder Dempster's favour.

Take, for example, the case of A.H., who had arrived in the United Kingdom in 1953 as a stowaway. Not long after A.H. arrived in the UK he found himself in prison for an unspecified crime. While in prison he applied for repatriation to Nigeria, presumably as a distressed British subject. Before his repatriation could be accomplished, however, he was admitted to Long Grove Hospital, Epsom, in February 1954, suffering from what was diagnosed as schizophrenia. As a result, his repatriation was temporarily postponed until 1956, when medical authorities finally cleared him for travel.

While an unambiguous assessment of A.H.'s mental state at the time of departure is impossible to obtain, there is some evidence that the authorities making his arrangements probably considered him to be in fairly poor shape, even by the standards of repatriated mental patients. Enquiries had been made prior to repatriation whether he could be admitted to a mental institution in Nigeria upon his arrival. This type of enquiry would be made only in a severe case in which it was considered unlikely that family would be able to take care of the patient when he arrived home. In Nigeria at the time, asylum space was restricted to only the most violent and dangerous cases, and repatriation of West African mental patients was usually predicated on the hope that they would be able to avoid further hospital care as a result of being back in friendly and familiar social surroundings. That A.H. was considered a likely case for admission to a Nigerian mental asylum before he even sailed for home is an indication that his case was quite severe and that he was at a heightened risk of causing difficulties on the voyage.

Despite his relatively unstable condition, A.H. sailed for home aboard the Elder Dempster vessel *Apapa* on 18 November 1956. The ship's surgeon had examined Hughes and found him 'quiet and reasonable'.[47] Nevertheless, six paid attendants, all of whom were government employees of Nigeria, accompanied him.[48] At 9:40am on November 26, A.H. stepped outside of the surgery quarters and headed towards the C deck of the ship, where, 'seeming quite cheerful and quiet', he enjoyed a smoke with a fellow passenger. As this passenger bent to set down the box of matches after lighting their cigarettes, A.H. took the brief window of opportunity to hurl himself overboard. The ship searched for his body for an hour, unsuccessfully. By 11:30am, the *Apapa* was back on course to its destination.

Official enquiry into A.H.'s apparent suicide produced no evidence indemnifying Elder Dempster or any of the passengers or attendants. In fact, the six attendants, as well as the captain, purser and ship's surgeon all gave statements to the police indicating that A.H. had acted without provocation or warning and that under the circumstances nothing could have been done to prevent his unfortunate death. Nothing in A.H.'s medical history or behaviour on board prior to his jump had indicated that he was a suicide risk. While the efficacy of the six attendants as potential guards or restraints on the actions of A.H. might be questioned, they clearly served as important witnesses who could corroborate the course of events in a way that absolved anyone but A.H. himself of responsibility for what happened.

The procedures that Elder Dempster set in place, therefore, seem to have served their purpose in protecting the company from being held responsible for circumstances resulting from its agreement to carry mentally unstable passengers. What the statements do not discuss in any way, however, is why a schizophrenic patient who required institutionalisation in Great Britain and presumably was likely to require institutionalisation on reaching Nigeria had been deemed an appropriate person to be discharged for the purpose of undertaking a twenty-two-day sea voyage. Thus, ultimately, the governments of the UK and the British West African colonies relied heavily on Elder Dempster to implement a repatriation policy that had no particular legal basis but which nevertheless dramatically undergirded the ideological foundations of the British Empire. Although such awkward circumstances necessarily created tensions, the British government and the Colonial Office needed the cooperation of Elder Dempster, as a non-governmental, private enterprise, to navigate the space between what was politically and medically desirable and what was legally allowable. While the link between state power and medical knowledge was strong, the secured cooperation of private business interests was also extremely important in enforcing imperial biopower.

Conclusion

Elder Dempster's cooperation with medical authorities and the Colonial Office over the issue of how to repatriate Nigerian mental patients contributed to the maintenance of a medical geography that reinforced notions of racial and cultural difference upon which the ideological justification of Empire depended for much of the twentieth century. Complicating the process, however, was the fact that the procedures governing how to repatriate these patients were a direct attempt to circumvent the medico-legal rights of individuals who were entitled to all the rights of British subjects, irrespective of their particular racial or cultural background. The inherent difficulties in such an endeavour illustrate on the one hand the symbiotic relationship that medical, governmental and private business interests shared in the imperial context, and on the other hand revealed the tensions between these groups over the issue of ultimate responsibility for the outcomes of their efforts. While it is a somewhat esoteric case study, it is hoped that this depiction of the role of Elder Dempster in carrying out the repatriation of Nigerian mental patients illustrates the extent to which the complexities of imperial medicine were by necessity broader and more intricate than the binary medicine/state relationship can account for.

In making this case for a broadening of perspectives in the history of psychiatry in British colonial settings, it is worth noting that existing scholarship in business history is remarkably consistent in its depiction of the relationship between Elder Dempster and the governments of the UK and its West African colonies. Overall, the impression is of a symbiotic but tense cooperation in which Elder Dempster and the Colonial Office relied on each other for the smooth operation of their various enterprises. Cooperation and collusion were commonplace. As Olukoju has recounted, when the United Africa Company threatened Elder Dempster's position by attempting to enter the shipping business in 1929–30, Elder Dempster lobbied the Colonial Office to interfere on its behalf to prevent the United Africa Company's move, which it did.[49] At the same time, in addition to serving as the primary shipper for private merchandise between West Africa and the UK, Elder Dempster also served as the exclusive mail and passenger carrier for colonial officials traveling between metropole and colony,[50] and granted the Crown Agents of the West African colonies discounts and rebates so long as they agreed to book exclusively with Elder Dempster.[51] During the Second World War, the British government essentially took over the shipping industry, allocating shipping space and priorities and requisitioning Elder Dempster resources as it saw fit for the war effort.[52]

However, the insidious ties between Elder Dempster and the Colonial Office also brought frustrations, disagreements and, sometimes, outright defiance. For example, Sherwood has shown that Elder Dempster frequently treated its black employees in ways that were contrary to British law, refusing them rights to transfer ships and failing to repatriate undesirable employees, despite a legal obligation to do so. The British government was irked by such behaviour on the part of the company but generally allowed Elder Dempster considerable leeway in its illegal representations of employee rights.[53] Also irksome to many colonial employees and policy makers was the requirement that they travel on Elder Dempster lines, even when they could obtain cheaper or faster service from other carriers.[54]

Despite the existence of such disagreements, however, it is clear in the historiography that the relationship between government and Elder Dempster was mostly mutually beneficial and predicated on a basic underlying principle that British private capital and British imperial governance should, at a basic level, reinforce each other.[55] Whatever their quibbles about rates and fares and laws, Elder Dempster, the Colonial Office and the Crown Agents all generally agreed on the importance of British control over the West African colonies, on the maintenance of a strong link between the role of the government and the commercial exploitation of the colonies and, perhaps most importantly, on the need for private shipping lines to maintain the desired corporeal, material and ideological ties between the motherland and its West African colonies across several thousand kilometres of ocean.

As I have argued in this chapter, these dynamics are also reflective of the role that Elder Dempster played in carrying out the medical procedure of transporting mental patients between the UK and Nigeria. On a basic level, the British government desired to rid itself of responsibility for non-native mental patients who were unproductive and ultimately a burden on the public resources of their host country. The desire to repatriate mentally ill Nigerians was also supported by medical theories coming out of colonial environments and adopted in the metropole that suggested that black Africans were not psychologically suited for European 'modernity' and that the greatest psychological stability for Africans came from being in their own 'primitive', traditional environments. At the same time, these patients, as British subjects, had specific rights that could not be denied in the ways that either governmental authorities or Elder Dempster might ultimately have liked. Disputes between government and company about the procedures, laws and liabilities of repatriating Nigerian mental patients occurred, but ultimately they found a way to cooperate. At the same time, the collusion between Elder Dempster, medical authorities and governmental officials worked to reinforce desired geographies of Empire – geographies that privileged white, European power and medical authority through the pathologisation and marginalisation of black bodies.

Acknowledgements

The research for this chapter was made possible through a Patrice Lumumba Fellowship from the John L. Warfield Center for African and African American Studies at the University of Texas at Austin.

Notes

1 The names of all individual mental patients in this chapter have been anonymised by the author to protect their identities.
2 Nigerian National Archives, Ibadan (NNAI) MH/59/S4/C6/1 letter from H.B. Shepheard, Welfare Officer, Nigeria Office, Students Department, London to Chief Secretary, Lagos, Nigeria, 20 January 1956
3 NNAI MH 59/S4/C6/2, letter from Wm. H. Shepley, Acting Medical Superintendent, Warlingham Park Hospital to Director of Nigerian Students, Nigeria Office, London, 29 June 1955
4 NNAI MH 59/S4/C6/2, letter from Wm. H. Shepley, Acting Medical Superintendent, Warlingham Park Hospital to Director of Nigerian Students, Nigeria Office, London, 29 June 1955
5 Megan Vaughan, 'Idioms of Madness: Zomba Lunatic Asylum, Nyasaland, in the Colonial Period', *Journal of Southern African Studies*, 9, 1983, pp. 218–38; Leland V. Bell, *Mental and Social Disorder in Sub-Saharan Africa: The Case of Sierra Leone, 1787–1990*, Westport, CT, Greenwood Press, 1991; J. McCulloch, *Colonial Psychiatry and 'The African Mind'*, Cambridge, Cambridge University Press, 1995; Jonathan Sadowsky, *Imperial Bedlam: Institutions of Madness in Colonial Southwest Nigeria*, Berkeley, University of California Press, 1999; Harriet Jane Deacon, 'Madness, Race and Moral Treatment: Robben Island Lunatic Asylum, Cape Colony, 1846–1890', *History of Psychiatry*, 7, 1996, pp. 287–97; Julie Parle, 'The Fools on the Hill: The Natal Government Asylum and the Institutionalisation of Insanity in Colonial Natal', *Journal of Natal and Zulu History*, 19, 2001, pp. 1–40; Lynette Jackson, *Surfacing Up: Psychiatry and Social Order in Colonial Zimbabwe, 1908–1968*, Ithaca, NY, Cornell University Press, 2005; Richard C. Keller, *Colonial Madness: Psychiatry in French North Africa*, Chicago, University of Chicago Press, 2007. For a compilation of a variety of different contexts both within and beyond Africa, see Sloan Mahone and Megan Vaughan (eds.), *Psychiatry and Empire*, New York, Palgrave Macmillan, 2007
6 See, for example, Steven Feierman, 'Struggles for Control: The Social Roots of Health and Healing in Modern Africa', *African Studies Review*, 28, 1985, pp. 73–147; John M. Janzen, *The Quest for Therapy in Lower Zaire*, Berkeley, University of California Press, 1978, as well as their co-edited volume, Steven Feierman and John M. Janzen (eds.), *The Social Basis of Health and Healing in Africa*, Berkeley, University of California Press, 1992. More recently, accounts of the relative abilities and inabilities of colonial state and society to impose biomedical norms and control indigenous bodies can be found in Nancy Rose Hunt, *A Colonial Lexicon: Of Birth*

Ritual, Medicalization and Mobility in the Congo, Durham, NC, Duke University Press, 1999; Julie Livingston, *Debility and the Moral Imagination in Botswana*, Bloomington, Indiana University Press, 2005; Stacey Langwick, *Bodies, Politics and African Healing: The Matter of Maladies in Tanzania*, Bloomington, Indiana University Press, 2011

7   See, for example, David Healy, *Let Them Eat Prozac: The Unhealthy Relationship between the Pharmaceutical Industry and Depression*, New York, New York University Press, 2004; Andrew Lakoff, *Pharmaceutical Reason: Knowledge and Value in Global Psychiatry*, Cambridge: Cambridge University Press, 2005, pp. 134–59; Charles Barber, *Comfortably Numb: How Psychiatry Is Medicating a Nation*, New York, Pantheon Books, 2008

8   See, for example, Dennis D. Cordell, Joel W. Gregory and Victor Piché, *Hoe and Wage: A Social History of a Circular Migration System in West Africa*, Boulder, CO, Westview Press, 1996; Francois Manchuelle, *Willing Migrants: Soninke Labor Diasporas, 1848–1960*, Athens, OH: Ohio University Press, 1997

9   I make no value judgment here about whether such individuals 'really' suffered from mental illness or not. The documentary records are open to interpretation, and the accuracy of psychiatric diagnosis is a fraught subject in the context of face-to-face consultation. Cross-cultural psychiatric diagnosis is even more fraught. See, for example, Roland Littlewood and Maurice Lipsedge, *Aliens and Alienists: Ethnic Minorities and Psychiatry*, New York, Penguin, 1982, for a detailed discussion of the difficulties involved in the cross-cultural articulation of psychological disorder. For purposes of this chapter, suffice it to say that British medical authorities were of the opinion that these Nigerians were suffering from mental illnesses.

10   NNAI CSO/26/06285 vol. I

11   NNAI CSO/26/03028 vol. IV

12   Oscar Gish, 'Colour and Skill: British Immigration, 1955–68', *International Migration Review*, 3, 1968, pp. 19–37

13   For a history of Elder Dempster & Co., see Peter N. Davies, *The Trade Makers: Elder Dempster in West Africa, 1852–1972; 1973–1989*, St. John's, International Maritime Economic History Association, 2000

14   Ayodeji Olukoju, '"Helping Our Own Shipping": Official Passages to Nigeria, 1914–45', *Journal of Transport History*, 20, 1999, pp. 30–45

15   National Archives of Ghana, Accra (NAG) CSO 11/8/16 letter from Alex Fiddian to G.A.S. Northcote, Esq., 20 September 1932

16   Sadowsky, *Imperial Bedlam*, pp. 26–47

17   NNAI MH/59/S4/9–10 letter from C.J. Maybe, Ministry of Health, Nigeria to D.S. Timms, Colonial Office, London, 11 July 1955

18   Matthew M. Heaton, 'Stark Roving Mad: The Repatriation of Nigerian Mental Patients and the Global Construction of Mental Illness, 1906–1960', unpublished PhD thesis, University of Texas at Austin, 2008

19   See Megan Vaughan, *Curing their Ills: Colonial Power and African Illness*, Cambridge, Polity Press, 1991; McCulloch, *Colonial Psychiatry*; Sadowsky, *Imperial Bedlam*

20   Correspondence between Elder Dempster and the Colonial Office on the subject of repatriating Nigerians makes it clear that West African governments already had legislation on the books for the repatriation of Europeans to the UK. See The National Archives, UK (TNA) CO/876/226

21   On tropical neurasthenia in East Africa, see Anna Crozier, 'What Was Tropical about Tropical Neurasthenia', *Journal of the History of Medicine and Allied Sciences*, 64, 2009, pp. 518–48

22   McCulloch, *Colonial Psychiatry*. Perhaps the best primary source on the subject is J.C. Carothers, *The African Mind in Health and Disease*, Geneva, World Health Organization, 1955, which provides a synthesis of available psychological and psychiatric literature on Africans at the time that the repatriations discussed here were in full swing.

23   Vaughan, *Curing Their Ills*, p. 101

24 M.J. Field, *Search for Security: An Ethno-Psychiatric Study of Rural Ghana*, Evanston, IL, Northwestern University Press, 1960, pp. 318–19; Raymond Prince, 'The "Brain Fag" Syndrome in Nigerian Students', *Journal of Mental Science*, 106, 1960, pp. 559–70, at p. 559

25 R.J. Still, 'Mental Health in Overseas Students', *Proceedings of the British Student Health Association*, 1961, pp. 59–61, at pp. 59–60

26 Cecil B. Kidd, 'Psychiatric Morbidity among Students', *British Journal of Preventive and Social Medicine*, 19, 1965, pp. 143–50, at p. 148

27 NNAI CSO/03028/S.978/1 letter from Secretary of State for the Colonies to the Officer Administering the Government of Nigeria, 23 August 1950

28 NNAI CSO/03028/S.1051/1 letter from Secretary of State for the Colonies to the Officer Administering the Government of Nigeria, 12 August 1952

29 NNAI MH/59/S.4/C.4/2 letter from Chief Secretary of the Federation, Nigeria, to Permanent Secretary, Ministry of Social Services, 10 January 1956

30 NNAI MH/59/S.4/C.27/3 letter from Consultant Psychiatrist at Long Grove Hospital, Epsom, Surrey, to Colonial Office, 7 October 1958

31 For example, in the case of M.S., a patient at Freirn Hospital in the UK in 1956, the patient refused repatriation, deciding instead that he would rather continue to convalesce in hospital in order to be released back into the UK one day. See NNAI CSO/26/03028/S.988/27 letter from Secretary of State for the Colonies to Officer Administering the Government of the Federation of Nigeria, 8 January 1957

32 NNAI CSO/03028/s.931/2 letter from Labour Department, Gold Coast to the Labour Officer, Lagos, 15 October 1945

33 TNA CO/876/226 letter from Elder Dempster to Colonial Office, 16 June 1950

34 TNA CO/876/226 letter from J.I. Loe, Passenger Agent, Elder Dempster to Crown Agents, 16 January 1950

35 This brought the overall cost of repatriating a single mental patient to the astronomical sum of approximately £180. Very few Nigerians could afford to pay such rates and, as a result, the government of the UK almost always footed the bill.

36 TNA CO/876/226 draft despatch from Colonial Office to Crown Agents, n.d.

37 TNA CO/876/226 letter from Ministry of Health to Undersecretary of State, Colonial Office, 24 May 1950

38 TNA CO/876/226 draft despatch from Colonial Office to Crown Agents, n.d.

39 TNA CO/876/226 draft despatch from Colonial Office to Crown Agents, n.d.

40 NNAI MH/59/S.4/13 letter from Colonial Office to the Officer Administering the Government of Nigeria: Gold Coast: Sierra Leone: Gambia, 30 June 1950

41 TNA CO/876/226 letter from Elder Dempster to Colonial Office, 16 June 1950

42 TNA CO/876/226 letter from Elder Dempster to Colonial Office, 16 June 1950

43 TNA CO/876/226 letter from Acting Governor, Nigeria, to Secretary of State for the Colonies, 19 October 1950

44 TNA CO/876/226 letter from Acting Governor, Nigeria, to Secretary of State for the Colonies, 19 October 1950

45 TNA CO/876/226 draft letter from Colonial Office to Crown Agents, n.d.

46 NNAI MH/59/S.4/20 letter from Office of Chief Secretary of the Federation to Senior Assistant Secretary (Education), Ministry of Natural Resources & Social Services, Lagos, 15 September 1955

47 NNAI CSO/03028/S.1088/4 'Details Concerning the Death of Mr. A.J.H.: Copy of Log Entry', 24 November 1954, p. 5

48 Two worked for the Nigerian Railway, two for public works departments, one for the Civil Secretary's Office in Kaduna and one for the Education Department in Lagos.

49 Ayodeji Olukoju, 'Imperial Business Umpire: The Colonial Office, United Africa Company, Elder Dempster, and "The Great Shipping War" of 1929–1930', in Toyin Falola and Emily Brownell (eds.), *Africa, Empire and Globalization: Essays in Honor of A.G. Hopkins*, Durham, NC, Carolina Academic Press, 2011, pp. 167–89

50 Olukoju, '"Helping Our Own Shipping"'

51 Davies, *Trade Makers*, p. 75

52 Davies, *Trade Makers*, pp. 255–71

53 Marika Sherwood, 'African Seamen, Elder Dempster and the Government, 1940–42', *Immigrants and Minorities*, 13, 1994, pp. 130–45

54 Olukoju, '"Helping Our Own Shipping"'

55 Although with sometimes drastically different value judgements placed on this cooperation. See, for example, Markia Sherwood, 'Elder Dempster and West Africa 1891–c.1940: The Genesis of Underdevelopment', *International Journal of African Historical Studies*, 30, 1993, pp. 253–76 for a particularly negative spin, while P.N. Davies, 'The Impact of the Expatriate Shipping Lines on the Economic Development of British West Africa', *Business History*, 19, 1977, pp. 3–17, at p. 14 argues that 'the investment which Elder Dempster generated and provided in its own self-interest had largely beneficial effects on the economy of British West Africa'. On the issue of the mutually reinforcing roles of imperial governance and capitalist shipping enterprises, see also Ayodeji Olukoju, 'Elder Dempster and the Shipping Trade of Nigeria during the First World War', *Journal of African History*, 33, 1992, pp. 255–71

Social disease and social science: the intellectual influence of non-medical research on policy and practice in the Colonial Medical Service in Tanganyika and Uganda

Shane Doyle

In scholarship since the mid-1980s colonial medicine has often been described as a key element in the imperial state's attempt to understand, monitor and control subject communities. Moreover, scholars have noted how colonial hagiographies emphasised doctors' intimate knowledge of local attitudes and practices, shaped by humanitarian concern and long service, extolled the technological mastery of the imperial scientist, and praised the power of the colonial state to transform communities, legitimised and facilitated by medical expertise.[1] These assertions and ambitions, however, were not always realised. Medical interventions were frequently shaped by racial or political rather than objective, scientific motivations, and their consequences could be destabilising rather than hegemonic. Moreover, doctors were not always blind to the limits of their understanding of indigenous societies. As colonial states matured, and medical officers' attention moved beyond the needs of European officials and the local servants, soldiers and police who sustained them, so their lack of knowledge of the underlying causes of disease among the wider indigenous population provoked increasing concern. Some conditions, defined as social diseases, demanded particular attention, because their incidence was recognised as being shaped by the imperfectly understood nature of local societies. This chapter will examine the nature of colonial knowledge, and the formulation of medical interventions, by focusing on colonial reactions to two social diseases in two neighbouring societies: sexually transmitted infections (STIs) in Buhaya in colonial Tanganyika and malnutrition in Buganda, the largest kingdom in Uganda.[2]

In particular, the chapter will consider the role played by non-medical academic researchers, who were affiliated to the colonial state, in shaping medical understanding of the context within which these two particular medical problems existed. Government anthropologists and a variety of social scientists attached to the East African Institute for Social Research, funded by the British Colonial Office, provided vital input and scientific legitimacy to the colonial medical departments' attempts to radically reform African sexual and family life. These non-medical experts encouraged clinicians to understand local behavioural patterns in terms of African reactions to universalistic paradigms such as modernisation or attachment theory, as well as tribal particularism. Significantly, this development worked against the liberal tendencies of many late colonial doctors, who were eager to separate disease susceptibility from broad-based assumptions associating race with certain behaviours, and instead continued to foster a tendency to pathologise African social life through generalised discourses.[3]

Orgies of drink and women: ethnography, morality and STIs in Buhaya

When British officials displaced their German predecessors in Buhaya, in north-west Tanganyika, during the First World War, they found themselves in possession of a territory with several unusual features. The introduction of the plantain or cooking banana a thousand or more years before had permitted the development of dense, semi-permanent settlements.[4] Descriptions of the villages that ran along Buhaya's eastern ridges, dating from the period of German rule, are characterised by an appreciation of the superficially familiar nature of this intensively cultivated landscape. Within Haya settlements surpluses were produced, food was readily available, paths were shaded and swept, huts were large and solidly constructed and plots were separated from their neighbours by tall, meticulously maintained hedges.[5] By contrast, the onset of British rule in 1916 introduced a new culture of colonial criticism and reformism which targeted not only local land husbandry but also Haya behaviour. In part, this new interventionism reflected a positive appreciation of Buhaya's economic potential. The young colonial state of Tanganyika, determined to wean itself off metropolitan subsidy as quickly as possible, saw in Buhaya a source of significant revenue. Early investment in coffee nurseries and a degree of coercion soon brought spectacular results. By 1923 Buhaya's coffee exports were already worth £113,387. By 1928 their value had more than quadrupled. Coffee was so well suited to eastern Buhaya's farming system that almost all the land that supported bananas was quickly intercropped with robusta coffee. The sudden prosperity that landholders enjoyed from the early 1920s had some unexpectedly far-reaching repercussions. Chiefly patronage became devalued, the transfer of resources to the younger generation was delayed and new inequalities within marital relationships began to emerge. By the mid-1920s these various sources of social tension had all become associated with one peculiarly emotive issue, sexual behaviour. This was because sex workers had come to rival coffee as Buhaya's most famous export. Anxiety about prostitution justified a tendency towards radical interventionism in the realm of sexuality that was sustained by evolving political, moral and economic debates right through to decolonisation.[6]

Ethnographers and officials alike associated the exceptional frequency of commercial sex work among Haya women with the new, coffee-related commercialism of Haya society. According to the anthropologists Southall and Gutkind, the enhancement of the material value of female labour inflated bridewealth to such a degree that husbands began to behave toward their wives 'as headmen rather than as lovers, keeping them slaving to make up for the expense incurred to get them'.[7] Colonial officials believed that wives, their sense of self-worth increasingly shaped by school and church, in turn demanded material recognition of the market value of their labour. The 'silk, perfume and high heeled shoes' worn by the mistresses of colonial officials and Indian merchants in the district capital, Bukoba, were reportedly coveted by rural women as early as the 1920s. Household heads' refusal to satisfy this craving for luxury supposedly gave unmarried younger men an opportunity 'by gifts of clothes and money [to] render the women independent of their husbands'. It is striking how lacking in patriarchal condemnation European comments on Haya sexual behaviour in this period were. According to the 1925 district annual report, women 'proceeding to Nairobi and Kampala rather than submitting to the old social order of things in Bukoba' was inevitable, given male elders' greed, the inequitable nature of Haya marriage and the 'idleness and promiscuous immorality of the younger men'.[8]

However, the assumption that declining marital stability and fidelity had made sexually transmitted diseases endemic within Buhaya limited the sympathy felt for women. STIs were blamed for both the low productivity and the low fertility of the Haya, so that sexual misconduct was viewed explicitly as a threat to tax revenues. Given that Buhaya was one of only a handful of areas of significant economic development in interwar Tanganyika, inaction was not an option.[9]

This tendency towards interventionism which characterised the British colonial state in Buhaya, then, was partly based on the significance of the district's coffee industry, and partly derived from the perception that the Haya were undermining not only their own health but also that of the fragile colonial economy as a result of their sexual immorality and the exceptionally high prevalence of STIs. In the early 1920s Buhaya, like societies across the border in Uganda, was described by local Europeans as suffering from nearly universal syphilitic infection.[10] Whereas medical opinion grew much more cautious in Uganda from the mid-1920s, in Buhaya the belief that STIs were so prevalent that the population faced possible extinction was still expressed into the mid-1950s.[11] In part this simply reflected the relative absence of external critical analysis of medical policy, but the sense that the Haya suffered extreme levels of STI infection did have some statistical basis, even if the data recorded were of uneven reliability. In 1925 syphilis accounted for 31 per cent and gonorrhoea for 7 per cent of all out-patient diagnoses at Bukoba hospital. In 1928 42 per cent of all cases treated in Buhaya's many dispensaries and dressing stations were diagnosed as syphilis, three and a half times greater than the national average. The number of syphilis cases per capita also rose significantly between the wars. In 1938 Bukoba treated by far the largest number of STI patients of all the hospitals in the Territory, accounting for a sixth of Tanganyika's gonorrhoea cases and a tenth of all syphilis cases. In the early 1940s a quarter of women attending ante-natal clinics had strongly positive Kahn tests for syphilis, and one in five Haya recruits for military service were diagnosed as suffering from gonorrhoea. A third of all operations at Bukoba hospital were external urethrotomies to relieve strictures that were assumed to result from untreated gonorrhoea.[12] The British Army's venereologist in East Africa encountered 'an amazing amount of gonorrhoea and many phagedenic penile lesions' in Bukoba in 1944, the latter probably a reference to chancroid. In the early 1950s the East African Medical Survey, having adopted extremely careful diagnostic methods, found that 6.8 per cent of men in three communities surveyed had gonorrhoea, and 17.1 per cent of the entire population surveyed had strongly positive Kahn test results.[13] It seems clear that STIs were a much greater problem here than in most East African societies.

For European officials, sex work was a symptom of a larger malaise affecting Haya society. In 1947 Elspeth Huxley, inspired by Goethe's tale of 'die Geister, die ich rief', toured East Africa in order to investigate how indigenous societies had responded to the uncontrollable 'sorcerer's magic' of European culture and technology. Whereas much of the region seemed to her doomed to dearth and desertification, Buhaya's banana–coffee permaculture had brought about a utopia of stable incomes, relative ease and food security. 'The Bahaya[14] seem to have achieved, in large measure, that state towards which our own society is so painfully struggling: the enjoyment of long hours, indeed weeks, of leisure, freedom from fear and want, and the satisfaction of material needs at the expense of the minimum of effort.' While drawing on the Arcadian literary tradition in her description of Buhaya, Huxley's writing also made deliberate reference to contemporary claims about what could be achieved by the new technocratic, welfarist developmentalism of the post-war Empire. But Bukoba's district administration, also employing ancient and modern tropes, corrected her assumption that the Haya had already entered the brave new world which was proving so difficult for the post-war government at home to create. Combining conservative scepticism about the character-weakening effect of welfare with long-established racial preconceptions, officials reminded Huxley that one of William Beveridge's five giants obstructing social reconstruction was idleness, and warned of the degrading consequences of leisure on the African psyche. 'This happy state, at least in their soft tropical climate, seems to have corroded their will to work and rotted away their self-respect and morals.' The Haya were the victims of '"too much prosperity"'.[15]

Throughout Africa, the sense that 'civilisation' and modernity were undermining social and moral structures was commonplace in the writing of administrators, missionaries and psychiatrists.[16] New colonial states everywhere had argued that Africans should be coerced into the cash economy by universal taxation and, if necessary, forced labour, justified by the assumption that there existed a reservoir of under-utilised labour within African societies, where women seemed to do most of the work.[17] By the mid-colonial period the destabilising effects of such innovations were the subject of much concern. In some parts of the continent, among the Bemba for example, monetisation itself was thought by observers to have undermined key aspects of local economic and social structures.[18] Colonial-era criticisms of, or concerns about, African prosperity, though, were not so common. The Haya were distinctive because their morally enervating idleness was viewed as a product of the low labour demands associated with both their traditional food staple and their new cash crop. Efficiency, so valued by Europeans when justifying colonial development and governance, was, it seems, inappropriate for Africans.

District reports had defined immorality as a by-product of rising cash income and indolence as early as 1925. The response to Huxley's admiring comments in 1947 were rehearsed many times over the years. Haya were regularly criticised for refusing to grow their coffee in the textbook manner, to monocrop or to mulch neatly. The same, frustrating lack of faith in European expertise was displayed in their rejection of colonial agronomists' advice on how to treat banana weevil, nematodes and panama disease, in the belief, largely correct, it now seems, that the declining productivity of their staple plantain crop was caused by colonial policies in the first place, and that the treatments on offer only made matters worse. Above all, they refused to put more land under coffee once its natural limit in the long-established villages of the eastern ridges was reached in the mid-1930s. Europeans were outraged that young men seemingly preferred to wait around in eastern Buhaya to inherit their fathers' plots rather than open up new coffee farms of their own. As early as 1932 colonial commentators had become convinced that the eastern ridges had reached their carrying capacity, and that young men were unable to marry while they waited for their inheritance. Officials, themselves self-sacrificing overseas servants of a colonising society, despaired that young Haya men rejected the opportunity to marry and move out west to the empty, fertile lands around Lake Ikimba, in favour of the seductive pleasures of the village. This lack of pioneering spirit, further evidence of the moral weakness of the Haya, was so aggravating because the stagnation of Bukoba's coffee production undermined not only the development of Tanganyika as a whole, but officials' own career progression.[19] In 1935, at its peak, a quarter of the coffee produced in East Africa came from Buhaya. Soon, though, optimism that the Haya would drag the rest of Tanganyika out of backwardness dissipated, and successive district reports bemoaned local resistance to scientific farming methods and declining tax revenues.[20] Buhaya's densely cultivated villages, the most productive land in Tanganyika, discomforted the officials who served the British colonial state. To them, the rotting mulch and humid shade, the high hedges and twisting paths, symbolised darkness and corruption, and provided a perfect environment for the nurturing of sexual affairs.[21]

Buhaya remained one of colonial Tanganyika's showcase districts, but its prosperity, literacy and political sophistication disturbed many of the officials who actually worked there. Bukoba was regarded as a 'difficult' place to govern. One administrator complained that its 'complex, vociferous and mass-educated population' was interested in only two issues, education and STIs, and observed that 'they suffer from both'. The tone of the memoirs of another district commissioner, Tim Harris, darkened in the chapter entitled 'Bukoba – the ultimate test'. Though forewarned of 'the never-satisfied ambitions and prideful sloth of the Bahaya as a tribe', he nonetheless found that 'the unremitting tension in Bukoba, coupled with the volume of work and the long hours of argument ... bred in me a near-paranoia'. Fatigue and frustration were the lot of Bukoba administrators, their creative energy dissipated in the adjudication of court appeals. A quarter of Haya adult males were involved in legal disputes in any one year. That such enthusiasm for the law was attributed by district officers to the Haya's misuse of their education, wealth and free time, rather than being taken as a mark of support for the *pax Britannica*, is indicative of the nature of colonial rule.[22]

In 1938, in response to requests from Buhaya's district administration and medical officer that some action be taken in response to the apparent threat of depopulation, three of Tanganyika's most experienced ethnographers were charged with investigating Haya sub-fertility. The leader of the team, Arthur Culwick, was regarded as one of the colonial administration's experts in ethnography and native affairs. His wife, Geraldine, who had studied anthropology at Oxford and had subsequently acquired expertise in nutrition and demography, accompanied him.[23] The third member of the team was Hans Cory, the Tanganyika administration's full-time anthropologist, who was believed to have an unparalleled understanding of the workings of African societies.

Cory and the Culwicks, on the basis of large-scale surveys, a study of local administrative and medical records and extensive interviewing, confirmed the local perception that 'The Bahaya are threatened with extinction as the result of venereal disease.'[24] Hans Cory explained the dissipation of Haya males in clichéd terms, their cultural integrity having been lost with their twin roles of herder and warrior. 'Because of the pacification of the country by the Europeans and the advent of rinderpest the men lost the purpose of their life and with it the concrete basis of their tribal customs and institutions.' Arthur Culwick too held that the 'breaking up of Bantu society' explained Buhaya's crisis of masculinity and morality, but, drawing on a larger concern about detribalisation, explicitly blamed social collapse on the very nature of colonial rule. As he saw it, traditional forms of discipline had been undermined by European libertarianism and the atomising, degrading economic independence provided by cash cropping. Indirect rule had permitted local chiefs to deflect European guidance through 'passive resistance and courteous obstruction', causing Haya to mock 'our administration as effete and incapable of even making the most highly paid native official do any work'. The result was 'the complete breakdown of sexual morality in the tribe. The Bahaya could hardly achieve a greater degree of promiscuity if they tried.' Haya wives, regarded 'as an agricultural machine and a domestic drudge' by their 'drunken, lazy and generally dissolute' menfolk, had quite reasonably chosen a life of prostitution. For Culwick, these women symbolised the corrupting, deracinating nature of colonial capitalism: they 'sell themselves in Bukoba during the coffee season and then migrate to Mwanza or Uganda for the cotton season'. The sexual freedom and endemic STIs which resulted had caused 'a much greater degree of neurosis than I have seen in any other tribe', and contributed to Bukoba's notorious difficulty as an administrative posting. Freedom from compulsion had made Haya men unruly subjects as well as bad husbands. Culwick's solution was to force the Haya to control sexual misbehaviour within their communities. He was 'unable to see that any able-bodied man has any right whatsoever to fritter away his life in an orgy of drink and women', and advocated coercion not only to improve public health and morality but also because it would, he believed, bring 'beneficial psychological changes ... which would make the tribe much easier to deal with'.[25]

Cory, instructed by Culwick to work out the details of the programme of compulsion, in late 1938 proposed the establishment of highly intrusive village-level societies or *viama*. These would facilitate the distribution of moral propaganda, the organisation of STI testing and treatment and the introduction of improving entertainment. Primarily, though, they would 'separate the healthy from the sick', with *viama* membership dependent on a negative STI test. Members would wear a badge, inform on neighbours who were infected with STIs and agree not to pay or receive money for sex. The real target of the campaign would be 'the worst offenders, the prostitute and the men of similar character. These mobile incubators of bacilli have to be rendered innocuous as soon as possible.' Cory anticipated that isolation and harassment would prompt 'a lot of the village beauties [to] emigrate', so he planned to establish quarantine stations at Bukoba port and the Uganda border where all female travellers would undergo examination and treatment for STIs.[26]

Cory and Culwick's proposals came to nothing in the short term. Culwick's condemnation of indirect rule and cash cropping was unlikely to win central government approval. However, when the 1948 census showed that Buhaya was one of the few areas in East Africa whose population had failed to increase since 1931, its district commissioner argued that this confirmed 'the trend foretold by Culwick ... the population is rapidly disappearing due to VD [venereal disease], prostitution and the general break-up of family life'.[27]

In response to these repeated warnings of imminent demographic collapse, Tanganyika's government requested that the newly established East African Medical Survey (EAMS) select Buhaya as one of its survey sites. The EAMS obliged, keen to understand why the Haya had not responded appropriately to the opportunities offered by colonial development. 'Here we have a productive area with a high rainfall, much money from cash crops, with available all the advantages of civilization, e.g. good educational facilities, first-class medical care and attention with a good general hospital, and readily available expert advice on agricultural, veterinary and other matters, with a central thoroughly efficient administration in command. And yet the tribe is dying.' The explanation, once again, was idleness and immorality. While the survey's 1953 annual report noted that there was no correlation between the results of STI tests and fertility levels, blaming high levels of divorce for Haya sub-fertility, the final EAMS report in 1954 returned to familiar ground. 'Extra-marital intercourse' and consequent infection with gonorrhoea were hypothesised to be the primary causes of the low reproduction rate. Only when the Haya were shown 'the evil of their ways' might their demographic problems be resolved.[28]

That the EAMS recommendation that Buhaya required a programme of intensive STI treatment and reproductive health information would be acted upon was far from inevitable. Colonial governments were wary of interfering in the realm of sexuality, and across the border in Uganda coercive interventions had drawn such embarrassing attention from London that STI policy there had become distinctly low key by the 1950s. Several factors combined to ensure that the EAMS's reports were put into effect.

Most obviously the enthusiasm of the medical department and of the colonial and chiefly administrations for an aggressive response to the STI problem in Buhaya was shaped by the exceptional prominence of sexually transmitted infections within the medical statistics. In addition, the belief that many Haya were unaware that gonorrhoea was transmitted sexually gave impetus to plans for disease control. Public health campaigns that focused primarily on correcting misinformation were always considered to have a reasonable likelihood of success.[29] Just as important, Tanganyika's medical department had already provided a model for the mass eradication of treponemal disease in the form of its yaws control programme, which treated 137,112 people in 1930 alone.[30] The potential of mass compulsory STI treatment on a local scale was recognised within the Tanganyika administration during the Second World War, moreover. In 1943 the director of medical services announced that it was 'the intention of this Department to carry out after the war campaigns against special diseases in selected areas of heaviest incidence, e.g. against VD in Bukoba'. Wartime experience had demonstrated the advantages of compulsory STI treatment within a captive population.[31]

Haya opinion had also begun to demand radical intervention to control STIs. Haya leaders put the district administration under intense pressure during the late 1940s to improve the medical treatment of STIs and to prevent Haya women from leaving for the cities. The official colonial response that STIs were social diseases which required reform within Haya society, and that freedom of movement was guaranteed for all subjects, was interpreted as a 'deliberate policy designed to reduce the population of the District'. Local administrators, evidently influenced by the Culwicks' suggestion that the healthy and sick should be segregated and that all who were ill should be compelled to complete a full course of treatment, were sympathetic, but constrained by central policy.[32] Tensions built as the STI issue became caught up with a wider debate about the use of Buhaya's coffee cess, a development tax which the colonial state had consistently employed to encourage the Haya to improve their techniques of coffee cultivation. As this involved more work with no immediate returns, the policy was deeply unpopular. The arrival of the EAMS offered the district administration a way out of the impasse. The pilot scheme's success convinced the Haya that the mass use of penicillin could eradicate gonorrhoea and syphilis. The district commissioner hoped that the use of the coffee cess to cover the high cost of such a programme would cause the Haya to take greater responsibility for their own health and reform their sexual behaviour. 'If not, the Haya would learn at their own expense that a purely medical approach will not work, and they would in future have only themselves, instead of government, to blame.' At the very least, a programme on such a scale would require the upgrading of all medical services in the district, so that the health and efficiency of the Haya would inevitably improve.[33]

The proposed campaign quickly took shape, partly because of the support of the EAMS. It seems that the EAMS offered at least implicit support to the concept of mass compulsory treatment because its medical researchers, like Cory and the Culwicks before it, believed that while prostitution had to be controlled, in general terms women were the victims of Buhaya's STI problem. As one of the project leaders remembered 'the men spent most of their time womanizing and drinking ... The women were made to do all the work ... All the revenue from the coffee went to the husband ... It is not surprising that several of the women revolted at such treatment and ran away.' Most female infections were believed to stem from their husbands' infidelity, and, due to the difficulty of diagnosing gonorrhoea in women, the disease had typically already damaged the female reproductive system by the time women sought treatment, if they did so at all.[34] A voluntaristic campaign, then, would leave most female sufferers untreated.

The success of the STI control programme lay in the decision to adopt a single-shot high-dosage injection of procaine penicillin as the standard treatment for both gonorrhoea and syphilis. The initial strategy was to treat all residents in the vicinity of each treatment centre who reported a history of STI infection or low fertility, dispensing with time-consuming testing. The medical teams relied on forceful persuasion, pressing local chiefs and missionaries to encourage attendance. As one participant recalled, 'They brought the medicine there, and people were being injected compulsorily. I saw it ... There was really meaningful propaganda going on, and the force behind it in the villages was kind of hand in glove, but chiefs were encouraging their people.'[35] Only in the mid-1950s, as the campaign matured, did testing begin to take on more prominence. The control programme in its early years was peripatetic, aiming to cure all infections in a defined area before moving on. By 1957 the decision to allow penicillin to be injected at all twenty-three of Buhaya's dispensaries saw the campaign settle into a routine of offering easily available cures for all new infections. The popularity of the STI control programme rested in large part on the decision to send the most able recently qualified Tanganyikan doctors to work in Buhaya. No longer dependent on outsiders with ethnographic expertise to provide expert knowledge of the social aspects of disease causation, the Colonial Medical Service instructed its own indigenous staff to use their social contacts to help bring down the prevalence of STIs.[36] These local doctors' view of the STI problem owed much to the analysis of previous writers such as Cory and the Culwicks, one advocating 'a complete change in the structure and customs of the tribe, first through the emancipation of the women and then perhaps by introducing a change in the economic pattern so that the young men share the work with the women and marry early'. Otherwise Haya women would continue to marry older men but 'get their satisfaction elsewhere' or become sex workers 'to lead a free independent life'.[37] But indigenous doctors like Charles Mtawali and Vedast Kyaruzi had a realistic awareness of the difficulty of effecting mass sexual behavioural change. Their focus instead was on the practical goals of persuading local sex workers to agree to voluntary registration and monthly doses of penicillin, and ensuring that STI control became part of a wider push to improve public health in the district, so that significant investment was made in female education, anti-malarial measures, water sanitation and the provision of nutritional health information.[38] Over the next ten to fifteen years, STI incidence fell significantly and, at least partly as a consequence, fertility rose sharply and divorce rates declined by a quarter.[39]

The role of the Culwicks' and Cory's reports in shaping subsequent medical policy should not be exaggerated. Their findings and recommendations were referenced by district administrators and by members of the EAMS, and the prominence of these native affairs specialists added weight to their proposals. But it is clear from the writings of Hans Cory and Arthur Culwick how heavily influenced they were by local discourse. There are striking similarities in the language used in Culwick's final report and the apocalyptic writings of local Lutheran missionaries in the same year. It seems likely, moreover, that the

Culwicks' assertion that sexual misconduct was the primary cause of population decline in Buhaya was at least partly derived from local European opinion, given that moral criticism was largely absent from their earlier work on depopulation in Ulanga. What Cory and the Culwicks added above all to Buhaya's STI debate was the authority of scientific expertise and apparent statistical proof. But the power of academic advisors, it seems, was greatest when their policy recommendations fitted neatly with, and were shaped by, local medical and popular opinion. The EAMS, for example, sought the assistance of the East African Institute of Social Research to analyse Haya problems of reproduction, but seems to have been little influenced by the findings of Priscilla Reining, one of the Institute's anthropologists. Reining considered that the role of STIs in causing Buhaya's demographic stagnation was exaggerated, and that the criticism of Buhaya's wealth and low labour input jarred with the development goals of the Tanganyikan state. She was disregarded. Discordant external expert opinion, it appears, could easily be ignored by medical practitioners.[40]

'The semi-sophisticated Baganda'[41]: malnutrition and modernity in central Uganda

It may seem surprising to compare STIs with malnutrition. STIs, after all, were diseases which were the subject of exceptionally intrusive and authoritarian medical interventions, justified by the danger to public health that they posed and their assumed origins in personal misconduct. But diseases linked to diet, like those associated with sexuality, were acknowledged to be profoundly social conditions, shaped by both entrenched custom and the cultural and moral transformation associated with colonialism, capitalism and Christianity. Controlling such diseases required an intimacy of knowledge of Africans' domestic and private lives that was considered unnecessary in relation to conditions such as malaria or measles. Acquiring such a depth of understanding of local attitudes and behaviours in Buganda did not require the kind of intense, project-like investigations seen in Buhaya with Hans Cory and the Culwicks' work in the late 1930s or the EAMS in the 1950s. After all, the Ganda were one of the most closely examined societies in colonial Africa. In the early twentieth century, a remarkable range of amateur ethnographies written by European administrators and missionaries, and self-descriptive accounts of customs and beliefs by indigenous intellectuals, constructed the Ganda as an African people who were exceptionally open to new influences from the outside world.[42] In the middle decades of the twentieth century a series of professionally trained anthropologists and psychologists, all interested in the Ganda's response to the forces of modernisation, produced a succession of ground-breaking works.[43] Though these social scientists rarely focused specifically on nutrition, recurring themes in their work were the state of the Ganda family and Ganda methods of childrearing. These issues formed the bridge between medical and social scientists who were equally interested in analysing the healthfulness of Ganda society as it came under what were perceived to be intense strains in the middle decades of the twentieth century. It is the collaboration that resulted that forms the focus of the second half of this chapter.

Once a showpiece of the British Empire, Buganda by the 1940s had fallen out of favour. European administrators complained that its famous Agreement of 1900 obstructed economic development, its *mailo* system of semi-freehold land tenure was blamed for creating a rentier class responsible for agricultural inefficiency in the countryside and squalor in town, and Ganda politics were increasingly dominated by populist, anti-colonial agitators who undermined the collaboration which had brought Buganda and the British wealth and regional domination.[44] Yet this period, which brought such administrative disillusionment, witnessed a flowering of medical and social science research. The war years had interrupted the normal leave pattern of the Ugandan Medical Service, with the enforced stabilisation of staffing facilitating new kinds of sustained study. In addition Kampala's Mulago Hospital welcomed a series of visiting research-oriented doctors, on leave or secondment from their military duties in the region. New ideas were introduced, permanent links were established with British hospitals and research institutions and a cohort of ambitious young doctors made plans to return on a permanent basis once the war ended. Many of these incomers were attracted by Uganda's long-established activity in the field of public health, but on their return sought to build upon this pattern of sporadic, top-down sanitary interventions by establishing a more community-based approach, aiming ultimately at the creation of a network of health centres.

Simultaneously, Britain's more intensive exploitation of African resources after 1945 was accompanied by investment not only in expanded medical provision but also in higher education. In particular the decision was taken to set up the East African Institute of Social Research (EAISR) in 1947, based in Kampala and attached to Makerere College, which was soon to be affiliated to the University of London. EAISR was established with the explicit aim of monitoring how East Africans were adapting to intensifying pressures to produce for the market, participate in new forms of political organisation and adopt Western concepts of law, ethics and attainment. Initially EAISR's academic staff were little involved with their medical counterparts.

The identification of malnutrition as the defining medical problem affecting the Ganda was entirely the product of Mulago-based research. Initially, as Michael Worboys has shown, malnutrition attracted the attention of colonial medical departments between the wars only due to the realisation that improved African diets would increase the value of 'the native as an economic factor'.[45] In Uganda the growing emphasis on preventive medicine during the 1930s, combined with deepening colonial concern about overstocking and the impact of soil erosion, resulted in the first nutritional surveys and the beginnings of local medical research into dietary imbalances. By the late 1940s, though, a group of talented doctors became convinced that *kwashiorkor*, or protein-energy malnutrition, was extremely common in Uganda. One, Hugh Trowell, would later write that *kwashiorkor* was 'the commonest cause of death in tropical Africa' in the mid-colonial period. The existence of the condition, though, was only generally accepted when atrophy of the pancreas, rendering advanced cases incapable of digesting food, was identified by Uganda's leading pathologist, J.N.P. Davies.[46]

Kwashiorkor, in the Ga language, refers to the illness suffered by an older child when it is displaced by a newborn.[47] Among the Ganda, this phenomenon was known as *obwosi*, and was associated directly with the maternal neglect of the older child, and more precisely with the abrupt cessation of breastfeeding that it experienced, consequent on the mother's falling pregnant again.[48] *Obwosi* assumed so much significance among medical researchers because of their awareness of the Ganda's unusual pattern of mortality. In the later colonial period, census results showed that as many children died between their first and fifth birthdays in Buganda as during infancy. In particular, Ganda children seemed especially vulnerable as they approached their first birthday and during their second year of life. This trait was first quantified in the late 1940s by Hebe Welbourn, one of the pioneers of community medicine in Uganda. Welbourn had initially come to Uganda as a medical missionary, but, put off by what she perceived to be the systemic overdiagnosis of syphilis, she transferred to the Colonial Medical Service in order to attempt to convince Ganda mothers of the value of preventive medicine. Her child welfare clinics grew in popularity and allowed her to conduct longitudinal studies of the progress made by young children in Buganda. The results of her work were first reported in her MD thesis of 1952, aptly titled 'The Danger Period during Weaning'.[49]

Welbourn pioneered the use of growth charts to track children's weight and height, finding that Ganda children were born small, grew rapidly up to the age of five to six months due to their unlimited access to breastmilk, and then their growth stalled, sometimes due to their first infection with malaria, but more often, she believed, due to the inadequacy of Ganda weaning methods. Babies were expected to eat a diet similar to that of adults, except even more carbohydrate heavy. For many small children the introduction of lumpy, indigestible foods, severely lacking in protein, coincided with their removal from their mothers in order to live with relatives. This cultural practice, she observed, was designed to help mothers and babies cope with the strains associated with a woman's subsequent pregnancy, but, among the peri-urban communities with which she worked, the difficulty of feeding a growing family in a primarily cash-based economy had accelerated the relocation of children. The psychological upset which followed, coinciding with new infections and exposure to inappropriate weaning foods, was, she believed, a direct cause of *kwashiorkor*. Welbourn's most significant finding was that the majority of the nominally healthy children who attended her child welfare clinics suffered from mild protein-energy malnutrition.[50]

By the late 1940s medical researchers based at Mulago had made a series of crucial discoveries which transformed understanding of the aetiology of *kwashiorkor*, explaining both why it seemed to affect such a large proportion of the Ganda population to some degree and why, in its acute form, it was so frequently fatal.[51] But finding an effective treatment still proved elusive, and, as Jennifer Tappan has shown, high mortality rates, highly invasive techniques of medical investigation and experimentation and a systemic failure to explain interventions adequately caused growing disquiet amongst many Ganda. Rumours of sorcery abounded, parents regularly removed their children from medical care before treatment was completed and, when riots broke out in 1949 due primarily to Ganda farmers' and workers' sense of political and economic marginalisation, biomedical researchers working on *kwashiorkor* were targeted. Medical research was suspended for a period, and when it resumed, a more cautious, culturally sensitive approach was adopted. This, then, formed part of the context which made medical researchers here particularly receptive to engagement with social scientists.[52] Further encouragement towards interdisciplinary engagement came in 1952. Crucially, the development of an effective treatment made the focus of new *kwashiorkor* research turn towards prevention. That researchers would devote so much energy to investigating the cultural causes of malnutrition was due in part to the publication of a report entitled 'Medical Research in the Tropics' by the chief executive of the United Kingdom's Medical Research Council, Sir Harold Himsworth. Himsworth, keen to integrate medical research at home and in the Empire, argued strongly against the environmental determinism that, in his view, had caused tropical medicine to be categorised almost as a separate discipline. His advocacy, and close involvement with Uganda's nutritional research, directed attention towards the social aspects of *kwashiorkor*.[53]

As a consequence, through the 1950s and early 1960s doctors in the Colonial Medical Service such as Dick Jelliffe and Hebe Welbourn worked collaboratively, and at times dialectically, with a number of social scientists. These anthropologists and psychologists tended to view childhood malnutrition as a symptom of a wider malaise, Africans' imperfect adaptation to colonial modernity.[54] This was a topic of general concern to British policy makers in Africa from the late 1930s as a series of strikes, damning reports of the destructive social impact of labour migration and revolts such as Mau Mau pushed colonial governments towards a policy of labour stabilisation and family reform. Labour contracts were extended; training and unionisation were encouraged, to a degree; key urban workers were granted a family wage and provided with family housing; and landholdings were consolidated. At its most extreme this attempt to remould African communities sought to break urban workers' social, economic and cultural ties with their rural kinship networks and to encourage the displacement of the extended with the nuclear family. Unsurprisingly, this attempt to reorient Africans towards a world where wealth was to be invested in direct descendants rather than distant kin, urban women would confine themselves to the domestic sphere and political activity would be deradicalised, had very limited success.[55]

Scholars attached to EAISR tended not to see their function as one of proposing specific policy interventions. Rather, theirs was a responsive, analytical role. And one of the recurring concerns of the late colonial period was the perceived weakening of Ganda familial bonds. Colonial officials, indigenous political leaders and local newspapers regularly complained about the growing instability of Ganda marriage, the rise in female-headed households, declining parental supervision of children and a concomitant increase in the frequency of premarital sexual activity.[56] This discourse shaped the research of a number of social scientists during the 1950s and early 1960s, whose conclusions in turn influenced medical analyses of the causation of *kwashiorkor*.

Social scientists' most significant contribution to the medical understanding of *kwashiorkor* derived from their work on the impact of fostering. This was a theme of particular importance for child psychologists in the post-war period, due to the influence of John Bowlby's work on how babies formed emotional attachments to their mothers, and thus how humans became socialised. Bowlby encouraged two researchers with interests in this phenomenon to examine it in non-Western contexts. Accordingly, Marcelle Geber and, several years later,

Mary Ainsworth came to Buganda, primarily because of Buganda's reputation as a society in which small children were routinely abruptly weaned and separated from their mothers.[57] Geber and Ainsworth independently observed remarkable physical and mental precocity among breastfed Ganda infants, whose motor, language and social skills were weeks or months ahead of their European peers'. Geber explained this phenomenon in terms of the relative lack of anxiety experienced by pregnant Ganda women and the 'loving and warm behaviour of the mothers' after babies were born. 'Before the child is weaned, the mother's whole interest is centred on him. She never leaves him, carries him on her back – often in skin-to-skin contact – wherever she goes, sleeps with him, feeds him on demand at all hours of the day or night, forbids him nothing and never chides him.' Both researchers, though, reported that the effect of maternal separation on the Ganda toddler was extreme. The resultant trauma and, in some cases, subsequent neglect by foster carers appeared to directly lead to a loss of these children's advanced physical state, and severe unhappiness, frequently demonstrated through anorexia or bulimia.[58]

The practice of fostering was examined not only by psychologists, but also by the anthropologist Audrey Richards, whose concern was with the social impact of the remarkably high incidence of fostering in Buganda. Her surveys suggested that a majority of Ganda children under the age of twelve were sent away from home at some point to live with relatives and learn good behaviour and clanship, a practice that had become more common due to marriage break-up, education, infertility and the economic power of elders in Buganda, who held most of the kingdom's land. Parents found it difficult to refuse requests for fosterage, and often actively encouraged it, hoping that a guardian's weaker emotional tie to a child would make it easier to impose discipline. Older children were increasingly sent to stay with relatives who lived in close proximity to a good primary school, while the ending of a sexual relationship commonly led to the rehousing of children, either because a single mother was unable to support them alone or because of the antipathy of an incoming step-parent. While Richards was careful to emphasise that many older children considered that being sent to live with relatives for several years had been beneficial for their character formation, and noted moreover that some children developed a close bond with their surrogate parents, her findings overall added to the sense that trauma was a common feature of Ganda childhood. Even where children were not sent or taken away from their mothers, social scientists argued that their psychological state was still often disturbed by the absence of a father figure. In 1957 the anthropologist Aidan Southall wrote of the strain experienced by urban families in

[142]

Kampala, due to endemic marital instability and the large proportion of households which were headed by single women. While a lack of male role models was hardly uncommon across urban Africa, according to Southall it was especially problematic in Buganda, due to the relative vagueness of its extended family relationships.[59]

A recurring theme in the work of Ainsworth, Geber and Southall was that the systemic inadequacy of children's upbringing in Buganda created a self-propelling momentum, so that damaged children grew up to be damaged and destructive parents. Researchers believed that the separation of a child from its parents and of a husband from his wife contributed to a range of social ills in Buganda: child neglect, the inadequacy of sex education, the supposed inability of many Ganda to establish enduring relationships of affection.[60] Crucially, these assumptions filtered through to medical researchers seeking to explain the severity of malnutrition among children. The paediatrician Hebe Welbourn, in a childrearing manual aimed at a mass Ganda audience, wrote that 'children who change homes several times ... never really trust anybody and seem to make difficulties in every home they stay in for long, including their own homes when they grew [sic] up and marry'. A few years later, in 1963, she noted that

> unfortunately it would appear that a large proportion of Baganda children do not establish strong primary maternal attachments. Indeed attachments of all kinds seem to be very tenuous. After weaning, the child may pass into a home in which there is no older person with whom he can make contact. He may be continually uprooted, passing from one home to another throughout his childhood. By adolescence he has very likely ceased to regard himself as belonging in any particular home. It is probably this lack of personal attachments, rather than weaning, per se, which presents the greatest difficulty in personality development of Baganda and which probably underlies such increasing prevalent social problems as promiscuity and marital instability, crimes associated with theft, and the revival of witchcraft and tribal religion.

Welbourn was far from atypical among medical writers in this period. Together with Fred Bennett and Dick Jelliffe, leading researchers into community health and malnutrition, she argued that

> all over Africa, increasing segments of communities find themselves involved in the process of rapid cultural transition.... The new town dwellers ... are usually quite unprepared for a life so different from their tight-knit village society. Overcrowded, substandard housing, an unfamiliar money economy, and especially disruption of rural tribal customs and regulations, tend to lead to increased incidence of illegitimate, unwanted or abandoned children, of venereal disease, and of prostitution and delinquency among juveniles.[61]

Doctors seeking to reduce the incidence of malnutrition in Buganda struggled to adopt a consistent line on the question of modernisation. Early writings tended to blame above all Ganda traditional weaning practices for the remarkable frequency of *kwashiorkor* in this society, noting that educated parents introduced their children to a wider range of solids than the mass of plantain and sweet potato that was typical fare in less 'modern' households. But as the 1950s progressed the focus of criticism shifted to two groups. One was referred to as the semi-educated, who supposedly aspired to a Western life-style and accordingly adopted bottle-feeding, yet lacked the standards of hygiene and income necessary to keep bottles clean and provide formula milk in more than 'homeopathic' quantities. The combination of under-nutrition and recurrent gastroenteritis that resulted was associated with particularly severe levels of mortality. The second group were single mothers, who had separated from the fathers of their young children and, unable to cope financially with the responsibilities of motherhood, weaned their babies prematurely so that they could be passed on to a relative at a younger age than had traditionally been the practice. Again, this was regarded as having particularly destructive outcomes. The early critique of stubborn traditionalism quickly morphed into one of a skewed or partial modernisation which corrupted both traditional and Western practices. This most familiar of social scientific concerns in colonial Africa survived through to independence.[62]

Conclusion

Medical policy is never developed in intellectual or political isolation, shaped purely by the research and practice of healthcare workers. This is perhaps particularly true of what can be termed social diseases, conditions where medical specialists require the input of other disciplines in order to better understand the context within which disease-causing behaviours emerge, and where officials and interest groups are especially likely to press for specific medical interventions. Certainly in Buhaya popular outrage and political leaders' sense of self-preservation helped ensure that the EAMS recommendations of the 1950s were acted upon. In Buganda, medical responses to malnutrition during the colonial period were shaped not just by the interests of a range of medical actors and funders, including the World Health Organization, UNICEF and the Medical Research Council , but also by the findings of a cohort of anthropologists and psychologists, and by Buganda's royal government, which passed laws aimed at restricting what were regarded as the most damaging forms of fostering. Social scientists, then, were not the only external influences on medical policy in these societies, and their counsel was ignored when it jarred with received medical or political opinion. But the collaboration between doctors and scholars from other specialisms could be significant, as it was in Buganda in the 1950s, when for several years local programmes against malnutrition concentrated heavily on the perceived problems of Ganda parenting.

Colonial contexts were particularly likely to encourage cross-fertilisation. Colonial governance prioritised stability and projected control, but it was profoundly insecure. The maintenance of distance between ruler and ruled obstructed the acquisition of knowledge of the desires and fears of the subject population, on which effective government depends. The quest for information tended to draw different strands of the colonial structure together, as seen for example in Lord Hailey's African surveys, or E.B. Worthington's studies of scientific research across the Empire. It also caused dependencies to seek to learn from each other, with Buhaya, for example, repeatedly mimicking Buganda's experiments in STI policy. This was no guarantee of best practice, however, for, as we have seen, post-war Buhaya adopted strategies that had been quietly abandoned north of the border.[63] While the ignorance of imperial regimes was in part a function of their limited resources, their corresponding advantage was that the scale of the state was sufficiently small for inter-departmental cooperation to be easily achieved, if the will existed. The district team, which required administrative and technical staff to meet regularly, was a common feature across British colonial Africa, sustained in large part by the simplicity of the state. Scale, along with shared backgrounds and worldviews, facilitated the interpersonal relationships on which knowledge sharing depended. Mulago and Makerere, medical and social science, were sited on neighbouring hills in Kampala, and their staff lived in the same neighbourhoods, socialised in the same clubs and often drew on similar liberal influences.

And yet, alongside the undoubted humanitarianism of the researchers who have featured in these case studies, the moralising tendency of the Colonial Medical Service in this region should also be emphasised. Medical discourse relating to STIs in Buhaya was remarkable for the consistency of its critique of Haya sexual attitudes and behaviour, whether the doctors involved were European or African, specialists or generalists. In Buganda, the early twentieth-century fixation with syphilis was shaken by metropolitan criticism of poor diagnostic practice, payments to chiefs who informed doctors which of their subjects were infected and the compulsory examination and treatment of villagers in front of their neighbours. By the 1950s Ganda sexuality had in theory become more a topic for analysis than for simple condemnation as social scientists were set the task of identifying the underpinnings of what was now termed dysfunctional rather than immoral behaviour.[64] Yet medical concerns about endemic malnutrition and systemic failures of parenting quickly drew upon long-standing critiques of Ganda sexuality, which was pathologised in new ways in the late colonial period, this time with the backing of science rather than Christianity. Now its excesses were attributed primarily to a malfunctioning family system, characterised by absent fathers, bereft mothers and rootless children. *Kwashiorkor* was thus viewed as a symptom of a more fundamental flaw within Ganda society, in which ill-considered tradition and destabilising modernisation undermined the socialisation of the young.

The severity of this wide-ranging criticism of indigenous society is surprising, given the Ugandan Medical Service's comparative reputation for social liberalism, evidenced by its early Africanisation, its recruitment of a number of South Africans whose community-focused health provision had jarred with the apartheid regime and its prioritisation of maternal and child health provision. Part of the explanation for this apparent contradiction seems to lie in the power of universalist theories which, for example, heightened expectations that Ganda would suffer a destructive form of cultural schizophrenia as they experienced modernisation, and that their children would be invariably traumatised by practices such as fostering. Many medical personnel, meanwhile, combined social liberalism with engrained assumptions about racial difference and, indeed, inferiority. It was not uncommon for researchers into *kwashiorkor* to wonder whether nutritional deficiencies on an individual or racial level accounted for what they perceived to be Africans' '"backwardness"', '"stupid[ity]"', or '"poor work performance"'.[65] But researchers were shaped as much by enduring preconceptions about local ethnic particularities as by the generalising tendencies of the social sciences and racial preconceptions. The dissolute Haya and the broken Ganda family were stereotypes which shaped the discourse of local Europeans and Africans alike throughout the colonial period.

Medical workers should of course take some of the credit for the failure of society in Buganda and Buhaya to fall apart in the way that some of the analyses indicated it would. Mass STI treatment and African doctors' cultural advantages in the development of prevention messages reduced morbidity and sub-fertility in 1960s Buhaya. Simultaneously, in Buganda mortality among infants and toddlers due to gastroenteritis and *kwashiorkor* was reduced dramatically. As Jennifer Tappan has shown, these successes were driven in large part by the critically reflective nature of medical research. Around 1960, the prospect of imminent decolonisation caused some colonial scientists to think about the wider logic of Africanisation. A conference was held in 1961 which examined which aspects of indigenous culture could be adapted to help advance the prevention of malnutrition. A new awareness of the role of under-nutrition and infection in the development of *kwashiorkor* prompted a shift towards community-based medicine, integrating social workers, community development specialists and agricultural extension experts. Multidisciplinarity now focused on prevention and alleviation at the local level rather than on the construction of grand theories of causation. A recognition that health education had been amateurish and shaped by external preconceptions resulted in a deliberate foregrounding of African field staff in new nutritional programmes, whose vernacularisation of the message of a balanced diet, *kitobero*, proved remarkably successful.[66] It seems that it was when significant investment in resources and research was combined with well-planned Africanisation that social diseases were most effectively challenged in this era.

Acknowledgements

This paper has benefited from the insights and support of Sunil Amrith, Felicitas Becker, Benedict Bigirwamungu, Emma Coombs, Asiimwe Godfrey, John Iliffe, Will Jackson, Charles Kahwa, Jesse Karugaba, Paul Lane, John Lonsdale, Gerald Lubega, Phillip Mbatya, Wilbert Mwandiki, Dr Mussa Ndyeshobora, Christine Ninsiima, Charles Otim, Jo Parish, Chris Prior, Syridion Rweyendere, Carol Summers, John Sutton, Yvonne Swai, and Hebe Welbourn; COSTECH, UNCST, the Red Cross, the Ministries of Health and the local administrations in Tanzania and Uganda; the AHRC, the British Academy, the British Institute in Eastern Africa, and the ESRC.

Notes

1   D. Arnold, *Science, Technology and Medicine in Colonial India*, Cambridge, Cambridge University Press, 2000; J. Comaroff, 'The Diseased Heart of Africa: Medicine, Colonialism, and the Black Body', in S. Lindenbaum and M. Lock (eds.), *Knowledge, Power, and Practice: The Anthropology of Medicine and Everyday Life*, Berkeley, California University Press, 1993, pp. 305–29; P. Curtin, 'Medical Knowledge and Urban Planning in Tropical Africa', *American Historical Review*, 90, 1985, pp. 594–613; S. Feierman and J. Janzen (eds.), *The Social Basis of Health and Healing in Africa*, Berkeley, California University Press, 1992; J. McCulloch, *Colonial Psychiatry and 'The African Mind'*, Cambridge, Cambridge University Press, 1995; J. McGregor and T. Ranger, 'Displacement and Disease: Epidemics and Ideas about Malaria in Matabeleland, Zimbabwe, 1945–1996', *Past and Present*, 167, 2000, pp. 203–38; Bertrand Taithe and Katherine Davis, '"Heroes of Charity?' Between Memory and Hagiography: Colonial Medical Heroes in the Era of Decolonisation", *The Journal of Imperial and Commonwealth History*, 42, 5, 2014,

pp. 912–35; M. Vaughan, *Curing Their Ills: Colonial Power and African Illness*, Cambridge, Polity Press, 1992

2   This paper will use Haya and Ganda to refer to the peoples who lived in Buhaya and Buganda, and also as an adjective to describe them.

3   For examples of growing non-racialism, particularly in Uganda, see for example 'British Contributions to Medical Research and Education in Africa after the Second World War', A Witness Seminar held at the Wellcome Institute for the History of Medicine, London, on 3 June 1999, http://www2.history.qmul.ac.uk/research/mod-biomed/Publications/wit_vols/44832.pdf, pp. 9–10; J. Iliffe, *East African Doctors*, Cambridge, Cambridge University Press, 1998, pp. 142–4. For discussion of the tendency to pathologise African culture, see J. Lonsdale, 'Mau Maus of the Mind: Making Mau Mau and Remaking Kenya', *Journal of African History*, 31, 3, 1990, pp. 393–421. For an example see J. Carothers, *The African Mind in Health and Disease: A Study in Ethnopsychiatry*, Geneva, World Health Organization, 1953

4   D. Schoenbrun, 'Cattle Herds and Banana Gardens: The Historical Geography of the Western Great Lakes Region, ca AD 800–1500', *The African Archaeological Review*, 11, 1993, pp. 39–72, at 50–3; B. Lejju, P. Robertshaw and D. Taylor, 'Africa's Earliest Bananas?', *Journal of Archaeological Science*, 33, 1, 2006, pp. 102–13

5   P. Kollman, *The Victoria Nyanza: The Land, the Races and their Customs, with Specimens of some of the Dialects*, London, Swan Sonnenschein, 1899, p. 68; H. Rehse, *Kiziba: Land und Leute*, Stuttgart, Strecker und Schröder, 1910, p. 2

6   R. Austen, *Northwest Tanzania under German and British Rule: Colonial Policy and Tribal Politics, 1889–1939*, New Haven, CT, Yale University Press, 1968; A. Culwick and G. Culwick, ed. V. Berry, *The Culwick Papers 1934–1944: Population, Food and Health in Colonial Tanganika*, London, Academic Books, 1994, p. 262; B. Larsson, *Conversion to Greater Freedom? Women, Church and Social Change in North-Western Tanzania under Colonial Rule*, Uppsala, University of Uppsala, 1991, pp. 92–114

7   A. Southall and P. Gutkind, *Townsmen in the Making: Kampala and its Suburbs*, Kampala, EAISR, 1957, pp. 82–3

8   M. Koku and M. Ngaiza, 'The Life History of a Housewife: Her Life, Work, Income and Property Ownership', in M. Ngaiza and B. Koda (eds.), *Unsung Heroines: Women's Life Histories from Tanzania*, Dar es Salaam, WRDP, 1991, pp. 85–108, at p. 92; Tanzania National Archives (TanNA) 1733/3:46 AB40, Bukoba District Annual Report (BDAR) 1925, p. 3

9   TanNA 1733/8 AB10, BDAR 1923

10   TanNA 1733/8 AB10, BDAR 1923; TanNA 1733/3:46 AB40, BDAR 1925 Bukoba sub-district.

11   Culwick and Culwick, ed. Berry, *The Culwick Papers*, p. 173 (quoting the 1937 annual district medical report); TanNA 215/2237, Annual Report for the Bukoba District for the year 1948; W. Laurie and H. Trant, *East African Medical Survey, Monograph no. 2: A Health Survey in Bukoba District, Tanganyika*, Nairobi, EAHC, 1954, p. 142

12   TanNA 1733/3:46 AB40, BDAR 1925 Bukoba sub-district; TanNA 215/77/B, BDAR 1928; Tanganyika Territory, Annual Medical Report 1928, TanNA Library; Culwick and Culwick, ed. Berry, *The Culwick Papers*, p. 173; Tanganyika Territory, *Annual Medical report 1938*, Dar es Salaam, Government Printer, 1940; Tanganyika Territory, *Annual Report of the Medical Department 1941*, Dar es Salaam, Government Printer, 1942; Tanganyika Territory, *Annual Report of the Medical Department 1943*, Dar es Salaam, Government Printer, 1944

13   W. Young, 'Extra-urethritic Cases in an African Venereal Diseases Hospital', *The British Journal of Venereal Diseases*, 20 1944, pp. 151–4, 143–4; Laurie and Trant, *East African Medical Survey*, pp. 119–34

14   Bahaya is the linguistically correct form of the name of the people of Buhaya. The term is now usually shortened in academic writing to Haya

15   E. Huxley, *The Sorcerer's Apprentice*, London, Chatto and Windus, 1948, pp. 191–3

16   McCulloch, *Colonial Psychiatry*, pp. 46–7; J. Sadowsky, *Imperial Bedlam:*

Institutions of Madness in Colonial Southwest Nigeria, Berkeley, University of California Press, 1999, pp. 99–100; Vaughan, *Curing Their Ills*, pp. 57, 107–8, 135. For contemporary examples see H. Gordon, 'The Mental Capacity of the African', *Journal of the Royal African Society*, 33, 1934, pp. 226–42; M. Field, 'Mental Disorder in Rural Ghana', *The Journal of Mental Science*, 104, 1958, pp. 1043–51; H. Shelley and W. Watson, 'An Investigation Concerning Mental Disorder in Nyasaland', *Journal of Mental Science*, 82, 1936, pp. 701–30

17 F. Lugard, *The Dual Mandate in British Tropical Africa*, Edinburgh, Blackwood, 1922

18 A. Richards, *Land, Labour, and Diet in Northern Rhodesia: An Economic Study of the Bemba Tribe*, Oxford, Oxford University Press, 1939. See M. Watts, *Silent Violence: Food, Famine and Peasantry in Northern Nigeria*, Berkeley, University of California Press, 1983 for a more recent discussion along similar lines.

19 Cf. C. Prior, *Exporting Empire: Africa, Colonial Officials and the Construction of the British Imperial State, c.1900–39*, Manchester, Manchester University Press, 2013

20 TanNA 1733/3:46 AB40, BDAR 1925; Tanganyika Territory, *Department of Agriculture Annual Report, 1932*, Dar es Salaam: Government Printer, 1933; G. Milne, 'Bukoba: High and Low Fertility on a Laterised Soil', *The East African Agricultural Journal*, 4, 1938, pp. 1–21, at pp. 14–15; TNA 215/1650, Lake Province Annual Report 1940; TNA 215/2237, BDAR 1948; D. McMaster, 'Change of Regional Balance in the Bukoba district of Tanganyika', *Tanganyika Notes and Records*, 56, 1961, pp. 79–92, at pp. 89–91

21 University of Dar es Salaam (UDSM), East Africana Collection, Cory Manuscripts (EAF.Cory) 104 Bukoba, H. Cory, 'The Haya Tribe and the Incidence of Venereal Disease, Bukoba 1938–48', typescript, p. 7. For further discussion of the frequently negative, and occasionally sexualised, depictions of African landscapes, see D. Hammond and A. Jablow, *The Africa that Never Was: Four Centuries of British Writing about Africa*, New York, Twayne, 1970

22 TanNA 215/2154, BDAR 1947; T. Harris, *Donkey's Gratitude: Twenty-two Years in the Growth of a New African Nation – Tanzania*, Durham, Pentland Press, 1992, pp. 235–7, 261, 266; TanNA 1733/8 AB10, BDAR 1923; TanNA 215/77/B, BDAR 1928; TanNA 215/2510, BDAR 1951; Larsson, *Conversion*, pp. 90, 105. Cf. Prior, *Exporting Empire*

23 The Culwicks had collaborated on one of the most important studies of population decline in interwar Africa, their analysis being based on life histories provided by 2,300 women. A. Culwick and G. Culwick, 'A Study of Population in Ulanga, Tanganyika Territory', *The Sociological Review*, 30, 1938, pp. 365–79

24 UDSM, EAF.Cory 239 Bukoba, A. Culwick, 'The Population Problem in the Bukoba District', 1938, pp. 7–9

25 UDSM, EAF.Cory 104 Bukoba, Cory, 'The Haya tribe', p. 1; Culwick and Culwick, ed. Berry, *The Culwick Papers*, pp. 124, 174–7, 228–9; UDSM, EAF.Cory 239 Bukoba, Culwick, 'The Population Problem', pp. 29–35, 41, 66. For a discussion of the colonial tendency to view social problems through a psycholanalytical lens, see W. Anderson, D. Jenson and R. Keller (eds.), *Unconscious Dominions: Psychoanalysis, Colonial Trauma, and Global Sovereignties*, Durham, NC, Duke University Press, 2011

26 UDSM, EAF.Cory 104 Bukoba, Cory, 'The Haya Tribe', pp. 9–19

27 TanNA 215/2237, BDAR 1948

28 East African Medical Survey, *Annual Report, 1952*, Nairobi EAHC, 1953, pp. 23–32; East African Medical Survey, *Annual Report, 1953*, Nairobi, EAHC, 1954, pp. 12–13; Laurie and Trant, *East African Medical Survey*, pp. 1–4, 138–40

29 TanNA 215/77/B, BDAR 1928; Culwick and Culwick, ed. Berry, *The Culwick Papers*, p. 173; UDSM EAF.Cory 21, Bukoba, District Commissioner to Provincial Commissioner, 10 April 1951; W. Laurie, 'A Pilot Scheme of Venereal Disease Control in East Africa', *British Journal of Venereal Diseases*, 34, 1958, pp. 16–21, at p. 21

30 Iliffe, *East African Doctors*, p. 40; TanNA 215/2237, BDAR 1948; TNA 215/2237, BDAR 1948; TNA, 215/2070, BDAR 1946
31 TanNA 31732, A.R.M. for Director of Medical Services to Chief Secretary, 18 October 1943, Minute 2, Yaws
32 UDSM, EAF.Cory 104 Bukoba, Cory, 'The Haya Tribe', p. 10; Culwick and Culwick, ed. Berry, *The Culwick Papers*, pp. 44–50; UDSM, EAF.Cory 239 Bukoba, Culwick, 'The Population Problem', p. 9. Cf. TNA 215/2237, BDAR1948
33 Harris, *Donkey's Gratitude*, pp. 261–5; USDM EAF.Cory 21, Bukoba, 1950–8, DC to PC, 10 April 1951
34 Rhodes House Library, Oxford (RHL), MSS.Afr.s.1872143, H. Trant, 'Not Merrion Square: Anecdotes from a Woman's Medical Career in Africa', p. 128; Laurie, 'A Pilot Scheme', p. 18; Laurie and Trant, *East African Medical Survey*, pp. 4–5
35 Interview (Int.) HL, Maruku, M, 6, 17 June 2000. Interviewees' names have been coded to protect their anonymity. Transcripts are available for consultation from the author.
36 Laurie and Trant, *East African Medical Survey*, pp. 135–41; USDM EAF.Cory 21, Bukoba, 1950–8, DC to PC, 10 April 1951; Int. HL, Maruku, M, 6, 17 June 2000; Int. JBK, Ijumbi, 11 August 2000, M; TNA/215/2700, BDAR 1953; TanNA, Acc.71 M.1/1 Medical general, Vol. 2, District Medical Officer to Provincial Medical Officer, Monthly report, West Lake, May 1957, 6 June 1957; TanNA/967.822.1, West Lake Provincial Annual Report 1960; TanNA/215/3449, BDAR 1957; Iliffe, *East African Doctors*, pp. 106–7
37 C. Mtawali, 'A Health Campaign in Tanganyika Territory', *Community Development Bulletin*, 2, 1951, pp. 54–6
38 Int. VK, Bukoba, 27 June 2000
39 Mwanza Archives, MISS/DN/53, Annual Report Bukoba District Council Medical Services, 1966, 30 January 1967; R. Henin, *National Demographic Survey of Tanzania, 1973: Volume II, Data for Socioeconomic Groups*, Dar es Salaam, Tanzania Bureau of Statistics, 1973, pp. 78, 32
40 P. Reining and A. Richards, 'Report on Fertility Surveys in Buganda and Buhaya, 1952', in F. Lorimer et al. (eds.), *Culture and Human Fertility*, Paris, UNESCO, 1954, pp. 351–404. Cf. P. Reining, 'The Haya: The Agrarian System of a Sedentary People', unpublished PhD dissertation, University of Chicago, 1967, pp. iv, 75–8, 131–6, 315–20
41 D. Jelliffe, 'Village Level Feeding of Young Children in Developing Tropical Regions, with Especial Reference to Buganda', *Journal of the American Medical Women's Association*, 17, 5, 1962, pp. 409–18, at p. 413.
42 The best examples of these genres are H. Johnston, *The Uganda Protectorate*, London, Hutchinson, 1902; J. Roscoe, *The Baganda: An Account of Their Native Customs and Beliefs*, London, Macmillan, 1911; A. Kaggwa, *The Customs of the Baganda*, trans. E. Kalibala, ed. M. Edel, New York, Columbia University Press, 1934
43 See in particular L. Mair, *An African People in the Twentieth Century*, London, Routledge, 1934; Southall and Gutkind, *Townsmen in the Making*; L. Fallers (ed.), *All The King's Men: Leadership and Status in Buganda on the Eve of Independence*, London, Oxford University Press, 1964; A. Richards, *The Changing Structure of a Ganda Village: Kisozi, 1892–1952*, Nairobi, EAPH, 1966; M. Ainsworth, *Infancy in Uganda: Infant Care and the Growth of Love*, Baltimore, Johns Hopkins Press, 1967
44 C. Summers, 'Radical Rudeness: Ugandan Social Critiques in the 1940s', *Journal of Social History*, 39, 3, 2006, pp. 741–70. *Mailo* derives from square miles, referring to the size of the hereditary estates allocated to Buganda's elite in 1900.
45 M. Worboys, 'The Discovery of Colonial Malnutrition between the Wars', in D. Arnold (ed.), *Imperial Medicine and Indigenous Societies*, Manchester, Manchester University Press, 1988, pp. 208–25, at pp. 210–11
46 H. Trowell et al., *Kwashiorkor*, 2nd edn., London, 1982, pp. xxv, 246; RHL MSS. Afr.s.1872/xxxiv, H. Trowell, 'Transcription of interview', 1982, 19

47 C. Williams, 'Kwashiorkor: A Nutritional Disease of Children Associated with a Maize Diet', *Lancet*, 16 November 1935, pp. 1151–2

48 RHL MSS.Afr.s.1792/45, M. Southwold, 'Ganda Conceptions of Health and Disease', Symposium on Attitudes to Health, typescript, 1959, pp. 43–6,

49 H. Welbourn, 'The Danger Period during Weaning. A Study of Baganda Children Who Were Attending Child Welfare Clinics near Kampala, Uganda', unpublished MD dissertation, University of Birmingham, 1952

50 Welbourn, 'The Danger Period', pp. 1–56

51 See, for example, J. Davies, 'The Essential Pathology of Kwashiorkor', *The Lancet*, 1948, 1(6496), pp. 317–20

52 J. Tappan, '"A Healthy Child Comes from a Healthy Mother": Mwanamugimu and Nutritional Science in Uganda, 1935–1973', unpublished PhD dissertation, Columbia University, 2010, pp. 78–105

53 For an excellent discussion of the larger story of kwashiorkor see Tappan, '"A Healthy Child"', pp. 99–109, 275–7. As she notes, environmental factors did in fact remain a significant area of research, given the emphasis placed on the structural limitations of protein availability in the Ugandan diet.

54 For a discussion of the evolving understanding of this theme within Africanist anthropology see A. Kuper, *Anthropology and Anthropologists: The Modern British School*, London, Routledge & Kegan Paul, 1983; L. Shumaker, *Africanizing Anthropology: Fieldwork, Networks, and the Making of Cultural Knowledge in Central Africa*, Durham, NC, Duke University Press, 2001, pp. 79, 155–6

55 See, for example, F. Cooper, *On the African Waterfront: Urban Disorder and the Transformation of Work in Colonial Mombasa*, New Haven, CT, Yale University Press, 1987; N. Hunt, *A Colonial Lexicon of Birth Ritual, Medicalization and Mobility in the Congo*, Durham, NC, Duke University Press, 1999; M. Shannon, 'Rebuilding the Social Life of the Kikuyu', *African Affairs*, 56, 1957, pp. 272–84; M. Sorenson, *Land Reform in the Kikuyu Country*, Nairobi, Oxford University Press, 1967

56 See S. Doyle, *Before HIV: Sexuality, Fertility and Mortality in East Africa, 1900–1980*, Oxford, Oxford University Press and the British Academy, 2013, ch. 4

57 M. Geber and R. Dean, 'Psychological Factors in the Etiology of Kwashiorkor', *Bulletin of the World Health Organization*, 12, 3, 1955, pp. 471–5; Ainsworth, *Infancy in Uganda*, p. 1. Cf. J. Bowlby, *Maternal Care and Mental Health*, Geneva, 2nd edn., World Health Organization, Monograph Series, No. 2, 1952. Ainsworth observed that weaning was not always as abrupt as it was reputed to be.

58 M. Geber, 'The Psycho-Motor Development of African Children in the First Year, and the Influence of Maternal Behavior', *Journal of Social Psychology*, 47, 1958, pp. 185–95, at p. 194; Geber and Dean, 'Psychological Factors'; Ainsworth, *Infancy in Uganda*, p. 420

59 A. Richards, 'Traditional Values and Current Political Behavior', in L. Fallers (ed.), *All The King's Men: Leadership and Status in Buganda on the Eve of Independence*, London, Oxford University Press, 1964, pp. 294–335; Southall and Gutkind, *Townsmen in the Making*, pp. 66–7

60 These issues were also matters of concern in 1950s Britain, and to some degree anthropologists' research interests may tell us as much about their own social preoccupations as about the African societies they described.

61 Ainsworth, *Infancy in Uganda*; Geber and Dean, 'Psychological Factors', p. 475; H. Welbourn, *Our Children*, Kampala, Uganda Council of Women, n.d. [c.1960], p. 36; H. Welbourn, 'Weaning among the Baganda', *Journal of Tropical Pediatrics*, 9, 1, 1963, pp. 14–24; D. Jelliffe, H. Welbourn and F. Bennett, 'Child Rearing and Personal Development in Africa', unpublished typescript in the possession of Hebe Welbourn, n.d. [c.1961], pp. 19–20

62 RHL J MSS Afr. s. 1872 146 Twohig papers, 'Malnutrition', memorandum written by J. Twohig, DMO Masaka, 1951; D. Jelliffe, 'The Need for Health Education', Report of a Seminar on Health Education and the Mother and Child in East Africa', Makerere Medical School, Kampala, November 1961, p. 1; Jelliffe, 'Village Level

Feeding'; H. Welbourn, 'Backgrounds and Follow-up of Children with Kwashiorkor', *Journal of Tropical Paediatrics*, 5, 4, 1959, pp. 84–95, at pp. 91–2. See Tappan, '"A Healthy Child"', pp. 178, 187–97 for a critical analysis of the limitations of medical assumptions that bottle feeding was, at core, driven by mimicry of Western modernity.

63 A. Hailey, *An African Survey. A Study of Problems arising in Africa, South of the Sahara*, 2nd edn., Oxford, Oxford University Press, 1957; H. Tilley, *Africa as a Living Laboratory: Empire, Development, and the Problem of Scientific Knowledge, 1870–1950*, Chicago, University of Chicago Press, 2011. See Shumaker, *Africanizing Anthropology*, pp. 69–71, 84 for a discussion of the Rhodes-Livingstone Institute's social scientists' imitation of the techniques and language of the laboratory, and their interaction with agriculturalists and ecologists. Its founder, Max Gluckman, argued that anthropologists should influence policy, be useful to government and contribute to development and public health.

64 Uganda Protectorate, *Annual Medical Report, 1952*, Entebbe, Government Printer, 1953; Women's Library, London, 3AMS/D/49, F. Webber, Colonial Office, to General Secretary Association for Moral and Social *Hygiene*, 30 October 1951, Uganda 1908–54; Int. HW, Bristol, 31 July 2008, F; A. Hastings, *Christian Marriage in Africa, Being a Report Commissioned by the Archbishops of Cape Town, Central Africa, Kenya, Tanzania, and Uganda*, London, SPCK, 1973

65 Tappan, '"A Healthy Child"', p. 118. Note that J.C. Carothers was admired for his humane treatment of the mentally ill in Kenya, yet depicted Africans as fundamentally immature, hypersexualised and incapable of logic or forward planning, due to the frontal lobes of their brains being 'functionally absent', the retarding consequences of endemic malnutrition and the damaging effects of African cultures, including childrearing practices. It should be assumed that social and medical scientists in 1950s Uganda would have read Carothers. Cf. Carothers, *African Mind*; J.C. Carothers, *The Psychology of Mau Mau*, Nairobi, Government Printer, 1954

66 Tappan, '"A Healthy Child"', pp. 133–4, 161–3, 219–27, 237, 243, 246, 272–7; D. Jelliffe, 'Custom and Child Health I', *Tropical and Geographical Medicine*, 15, 1963, pp. 121–3

CHAPTER EIGHT

Cooperation and competition: missions, the colonial state and constructing a health system in colonial Tanganyika

Michael Jennings

Patchy, incomplete and of varying quality over time and place: none-theless, since the late nineteenth century, missions and other faith-based organisations and religious institutions have been central to meeting the welfare needs of Africans across the continent, a critical component of what we might consider the public-private mix of public goods provision. As Anna Greenwood reminds us in the Introduction to this volume, 'colonial medicine' in Tanganyika (as with other colonies and imperial possessions) was never, and never could have been, solely provided by any one actor. The Colonial Service was neither unified nor unidirectional in its provision, and collaboration between the Colonial Medical Service and non-state actors was the norm. In Tanganyika by the 1930s, the claim to be at least attempting to meet the health needs of the territory could only really be justified (to the extent that it could) by recognising the voluntary role that actors in the form of missionary organisations were playing in running health services for Tanganyikans.

The model that characterised late colonial-period Tanganyika was one of public-private partnership. Having long acted as informally contracted health providers, by the mid-1940s missions became formal partners in the delivery of healthcare. In return for accepting greater government oversight of mission facilities and a requirement to meet state-set standards and targets, missionary medicine was to be finan-cially supported by the colonial state and granted privileged access to policy-making and policy-setting structures.

As Greenwood notes in the Introduction, such collaboration between colonial state and non-state partners usually reflected colonial self-interest, and the model that had emerged by the mid-1940s certainly did that. But it also reflected internal dialogues within and between mission medical providers as to their wider social role. In other words, the public-private (voluntary) partnership that was established reflected the coming together of two sets of strategic interests: those of the colonial state, certainly, but also those of mission medical providers. Moreover, the process of integration was one in which both missions and the administration engaged in, fought over and negotiated the final settlement in a way that confirmed the strengths and weaknesses that both possessed in seeking to establish control over that process.

But for anyone looking ahead in the early twentieth century, the emergence of this particular public-private mix of service provision, and the dominant role played in it today by faith-based organisations, would have appeared unlikely. How had missions, initially atomised and jealous of their independence (and regarded as such by the colonial state), come to formally partner the colonial state in providing welfare and social services that embraced education and health? This chapter argues that essential to that process was the emergence from the 1930s of a conception of a 'mission sector' which emerged within both missionary organisations and the colonial state, with implications for both that would last beyond the end of the colonial period in the country.

This chapter explores some of the dynamics between medical missions in colonial Tanganyika and the colonial medical department. Christian missions did not represent the only religion to be involved in healthcare, but their relationship with the colonial state and their status as major providers of health services created a space which they could legitimately use to create a politicised and engaged faith sector, capable of making demands upon the colonial government. Debates over the level of support that the state should provide for mission health services, conflict over specifics of policy and fears of government plans to establish formal control over medical missions helped to shape the emerging faith sector and the interaction between voluntary and public arenas.

Reinserting the place of the mission into colonial medicine in Tanganyika

Despite the growing literature on missionary healthcare, there persists a sense in much of it that missionary medicine is somehow different, separate from that of the colonial state. If not exactly written out of the historical narrative of healthcare in Tanzania, missionary medicine has been presented by some as an evolutionary dead end, making a minimal impact on the shape and structure of post-colonial biomedical services. David Clyde's official *History of the Medical Services of Tanganyika*, for example, written for the new government following independence, excluded the contribution made by mission medical services from any significant discussion. The 1964 Titmuss Report similarly rejected missionary medicine as an important factor in the evolution of the country's health services, noting, 'outside a very small circle these early endeavours by voluntary agencies made little impression on the health or health practices of the African population'. The real history of European healthcare began, the report noted, 'in 1888 with the period of German administration'.[1] Even Meredeth Turshen's account of colonial medicine in Songea District in southern Tanganyika similarly makes little reference to the mission hospitals, clinics and the doctors working there, seeing medicine and health services in the district as being determined by colonial state economic, social and political objectives. Where missions do appear in Turshen's account, they are as adjuncts to and collaborators with the colonial state. No differences are seen between the colonial state and mission priorities, ideological drivers and objectives.[2] The term 'colonial medicine' is used here very much as shorthand for colonial *state* medicine.

In reducing missionary medicine to either willing collaborator in the colonial vision of the occupying state or aloof outsider operating through a heady mix of physick and metaphysics, such accounts fail to capture both the realities of missionary medicine and the nature of colonial medicine in Tanganyika.

Colonial medicine, in the sense of European biomedical services within the colonial setting, was never the sole remit of the colonial state. For much of the colonial period, the landscape of European medicine as practised in Tanganyika, as in British colonial Africa more widely, was far more varied. It was a fragmented, disparate mixture of public (colonial state and services offered through the Native Authorities), private (individual private practice and health services run and paid for by commercial concerns) and private-voluntary (organisations providing services for both humanitarian and more metaphysical reasons). In terms of numbers, the state was never overwhelmingly dominant. Indeed, until the mid-1930s, and considerably later in some remote and rural areas of sub-Saharan Africa, missions remained dominant actors in healthcare provision; whilst in some countries private company services had exclusive responsibility over large swathes of territory.

The extent to which any particular sector (state, private, voluntary) dominated across time and between colonies varied. In French Africa, for example, the state loomed large as the ultimate source of social welfare for Africans. In colonial territories with significant commercial concerns (plantations, mines and other large-scale industrial activity), private practices for workers and worker families played a greater role. But in much of sub-Saharan Africa, with some notable exceptions, missions were significant providers of healthcare services for Africans throughout the colonial period, often having established themselves

[155]

as such before even colonial boundaries had been set and the violent occupation by the colonial state had begun. This was the case in Tanganyika. Writing of one area in southern Tanganyika, mission-owned and run 'clinics and hospitals provided', Terence Ranger notes, 'the sole effective medical facilities in Masasi district'.[3] The same could be said for many predominantly rural and often remote areas across Tanganyika and British colonial Africa more widely.

Nor were mission services simply filling in the gaps in colonial Tanganyika, as some accounts imply. Even before the emergence in the 1930s of an evolution towards a public-private partnership in the delivery of health (in which missionary services were formally incorporated into official welfare structures), mission medical services were regarded (even if not officially) as vital partners in making biomedical health services available to Tanganyikans.

Moreover, the transition to this formal partnership was more than a reaction on the part of missions to government policy, but reflective of internal parallel processes on the part of those missionary organisations. Certainly, as David Hardiman has written 'colonial medical departments became more interventionist, and more began to be spent on medicine'. But his assertion that '[i]n the process, they began to intrude on what had been regarded before as mission territory'[4] misses the extent to which missions proactively engaged in shaping the new structures and systems that emerged in this period in Tanganyika. This was no simple intrusion of the state into mission territory, but the defining of a new space in which both state and voluntary agencies co-existed. For missions had similarly undergone a process of reorganisation and redefinition of their relationship with the state, creating what in effect transformed disparate, individualised medical mission services into a more organised and coordinated (in policy terms at least) 'faith health sector'. Moreover, far from seeing post-war government expansion in the medical sector as an encroachment into their territory, mission policy – as expressed through the institutions established to represent this 'sector' – had been calling for greater synergy between mission and state services since the 1930s. Differences emerged over policy specifics and particular directions, but missions actively embraced a closer relationship with, and formal inclusion in, colonial state public health provision – before, even, the colonial state adopted such a position.

Speaking with one voice: creating the 'mission sector'

Even before German occupation and the establishment of the colonial state from the 1880s, missions had long established a presence in the territory. They provided healthcare and primary education; they offered training of adults in specific skills; provided (during the pre-colonial period) relief in times of famine, and refuge in times of conflict between the various political and ethnic groups existing in the region. From their first tentative steps in establishing a permanent presence, missions had gradually expanded their activities to include a range of welfare and social services. In the education sector, missions dominated activity throughout the colonial period. Whilst the mission was never the overwhelmingly dominant provider of health services to Tanganyikans, nevertheless, it made significant contributions in wider colonial healthcare too. From the very start, missions were far more than just the sites of Christianity, commerce and civilisation that the Livingstonean and Victorian imaginations of missionary enterprise had envisaged. But if by the 1910s and 1920s they had become, in effect, part of the mix of service providers, they could not be said to constitute a 'sector' in the sense of a collective identity, shared values and objectives and common interests. Reflecting the history of the expansion of missions in Tanganyika, spreading out from the littoral in the second half of the nineteenth century, mission stations remained isolated from one another. Lacking a single forum in which they could pool experiences and aspirations, belonging to different faith traditions and coming from a range of European and North American countries, missions operated as the largely individual, atomised units they were, competing rather than cooperating with their fellow faith adherents.

If missions faced few internal pressures to represent a more united front, there was also little encouragement from the colonial state itself. The administration remained determined to maintain strict control over policy and funding decisions, and consequently was reluctant to dilute such control through closer partnerships with non-state providers. True, the colonial state accepted the reality of mission-dominated primary school provision, albeit under government supervision and control. But as Ana Madeira writes in relation to the Belgian Congo:

> The missionary zeal in promoting vocational education was thus seen by the State as a practical economic investment in the sense that convergent ideology and consistent practice were saving the central government the trouble of having to spend a considerable part of the budget on financing education in the colonies.[5]

So too in Tanganyika, where, in 1925, at a conference called by Governor Cameron to discuss welfare services in Tanganyika, it was agreed that the colonial state would fund mission-run education services, in return for taking overall control of education policy and standards. And it did financially support mission medical services, albeit in a (deliberately) *ad hoc* fashion. Unlike its relationship with the education services, the Tanganyikan administration did claim to be the main provider of medical services in the territory, suggesting (rather spuriously) that its model of 'preventive' medicine was of greater value than the curative services offered by missions.[6]

Thus, if missions did not speak with one voice, nor did the government seek to work with missions as a 'sector'. As a result, despite missions making a considerable contribution to social welfare provision in colonial Tanganyika, there existed no recognisable 'non-state' sector pursuing common goals and agendas, sharing information and presenting a unified front to the government. The mission influence could not be ignored by the colonial state, but its lack of cohesion meant that in reality it held little influence over medical policy debates and discussions. By the 1930s, however, the pretence that the colonial state was the primary healthcare deliverer was becoming harder to sustain. The mission contribution in this area, fragmented as it was, was nonetheless critical in any claim to be meeting the welfare obligations of colonial rule under the Trusteeship mandate. Even where government hospitals were situated close to mission hospitals, the two often worked to complement, rather than compete with, each other. The Church Missionary Society hospital in Mpwapwa, for example, treated mainly women and children, whilst the government hospital treated men.[7] The state had effectively conceded maternal and child healthcare services to the missions, recognising the amount of work missions were doing in this area, as well as the innovation and appeal of such services in the areas in which they were situated.[8]

The scale of medical work undertaken by missions belied the colonial administration's claims that it alone was working to address the provision of biomedical healthcare in Tanganyika. In Shinyanga District, the government-run hospital and two government dispensaries treated 4,159 out-patients and 663 in-patients in 1926. The Africa Inland Mission hospital at Kola Ndoto, under the charge of Dr Maynard, treated 26,062 out-patients and 360 in-patients in the same year.[9] '[T]he major portion of the medical work' in Shinyanga, the District Commissioner noted, 'is being undertaken by Dr Maynard as a purely charitable work.'[10] In 1931, Dr Maynard and her medical team treated a staggering 69,826 out-patients, and attended 1,322 births in the Native Administration Maternity Home.[11] The Universities Mission to Central Africa (UMCA) saw 187,271 out-patients in its hospitals and dispensaries in Masasi and Zanzibar Diocese in 1936.[12] Even at the end of the colonial period, missions were making a substantial contribution: some 6,599,608 out-patients were treated at government hospitals and dispensaries in 1959; mission medical services treated 4,518,346.[13]

By the mid-1930s it was becoming clear to both government and mission leaders that the informal, personal linkages on which they relied for communication and cooperation were insufficient for the effective planning and delivery of key services. The lack of formal channels also prevented the easy articulation of a 'mission position', agreed to amongst mission representatives and reflecting common concerns, in relation to the major issue facing mission providers of healthcare services. From the perspective of the state, whilst this limited challenges to its policies from one of the few areas from which a strong and sustained challenge could have emerged, it also hampered government efforts to coordinate and work with missions when it could advantage the state to do so. The government survey of medical missions in 1936 in part reflected a growing awareness that the mission contribution was too significant to ignore. But missions had also grown more aware of the commonalities that bound them together as a group: a shared ethos and character, facing similar constraints and opportunities. In Tanganyika, mission leaders began the process of establishing more formal networks between missions, across denominational lines, in a concerted effort to increase the influence of the mission sector within the colonial state. The 1926 Le Zoute conference on the 'Christian Mission in Africa' had recommended the establishment of an international advisory board to 'assist the cooperation of medical missions with Governments': colonial states could, the conference avowed, 'count upon the missionary societies rendering all possible assistance to Governments in the forwarding of any particular measures of Public Health which it is desirable should be carried out'.[14] However, it was not until almost a decade later that such international mission policy was translated into meaningful practice in Tanganyika.

In 1932 the UMCA Bishop of Masasi wrote to all mission leaders in Tanganyika, expressing concern that efforts by government to work more closely with missions were being hampered by the lack of a clear 'mission perspective' on key policy issues. Mission views were 'so varied as to appear bewildering', he wrote, 'and the desire to give sympathetic support yields to disheartenment. The impression given is that we Missionaries do not know clearly what we do want.'[15] The remedy, Bishop Lucas suggested, was to establish a single organisation representing the mission sector, to enable 'common counsel' with the aim of 'attaining a common policy' to present to government.[16] In 1934, the Tanganyika Mission Council (TMC) was established as the fulfilment of these ambitions. Its membership consisted of the main Protestant missions working in Tanganyika, thereby frustrating efforts

[159]

to create a truly pan-mission representative organisation. The Roman Catholic Church had declined to participate, perhaps suspicious of a modernising instinct that it detected amongst the proposers of the idea, and already possessing a single organisational structure from which it could negotiate with the state on behalf of all its constituent members. It did, however, agree to participate on an informal basis.[17]

The creation of the TMC, which in 1949 would be renamed the Christian Council of Tanganyika (CCT), marked a new departure both for mission history in Tanganyika and for the history of welfare service provision in the country. It created a distinct mission 'sector', capable of speaking for a large number of missionary organisations operating in the country, negotiating and working with the colonial state as a sector rather than as disparate, individualised organisations. It marked the beginnings of what can be seen as the formal voluntary sector in Tanganyika.[18] By 1948 TMC membership included the following organisations[19]:

- Africa Inland Mission
- Augustana Lutheran Mission
- Church of Sweden
- Church Missionary Society
- Elim Missionary Society
- Mennonite Mission
- Moravian Mission
- Swedish Evangelical Mission
- Universities Mission to Central Africa.

The TMC was established as the broad representative organisation for all mission interests, including (but not confined to) mission engagement in social service provision. Meetings between government and the TMC thus included discussions on health and education, what missions could (and should) be doing and questions of how they were to be financially supported, alongside discussions on wider government–mission relations. In 1936, the Medical Missionary Committee (MMC) was established as a sub-committee of the TMC with a specific mandate to bring about 'closer cooperation between medical missionaries and the Medical Department of the Government'.[20] As a result, it became the main point of contact between the colonial state and missions for the discussion of missionary and colonial state medical services. The first meeting of the MMC, in July of that year, discussed 'the question of the relationship between the Medical Department of the Missions and the Government Medical Services'.[21] In return for being recognised as a formal partner in Tanganyika's healthcare service provision, missions might accept greater oversight from the state's Medical Department, providing reports, cooperating in training and accepting regulation of standards.[22] The impression given from the start was of a sector that saw itself, and wanted to be recognised, as an integral part of the territory's health services. MMC membership in 1937 comprised:[23]

- Augustana Lutheran Mission
- Bethel Mission
- Berlin Mission
- Church Missionary Society
- Leipzig Mission
- Moravian Mission
- UMCA.

The same year that the MMC was established, the colonial administration sought to better understand what scale of medical mission activity was being undertaken in Tanganyika. It called for data relating to in- and out-patients treated. The snapshot provided to the administration demonstrated just how much missions were doing (see Table 1). It was also recognition on the part of the administration that missions were undertaking medical work on a large scale. It was a scale of activity that was to grow over the next 25 years.

In 1951, the MMC, still a sub-committee of the newly renamed TMC (now called the Christian Council of Tanganyika), further institutionalised its function as the principal representative organisation of mission health services with a new constitution. To ensure that it spoke for the whole of the membership the MMC was to be open to all medical practitioners working within the mission sector. The heads of any mission with a medical service were to be invited to all discussions of medical policy, and minutes would be sent to all heads of missions with at least one medical practitioner.[24] Such measures helped to entrench the MMC as the legitimate and, more importantly, sole voice of medical mission. The following year, in recognition that the role of the MMC had grown beyond the original Protestant mission membership, the organisation was renamed the Medical Mission Advisory Committee (MMAC), henceforth to act as the 'representative of all Mission Medical opinion in Tanganyika, and should in that capacity be consulted and should advise on matters of Government policy affecting Mission Medical work', operating independently from the organisational structures of the CCT.[25]

At the national level, the efforts to create a more unified mission response were broadly welcomed by all missions. The MMC was

Table 1 Summary of medical missionary work in 1936 for selected Protestant missions*

Mission	Out-patients	Hospitals	Dispensaries
Augustana Lutheran Mission, Kiomboi	88,770	2	3
Bethel Mission, Bukoba	14,100	2	5
Moravian Mission, Tabora	11,500	1	3
Leipzig Lutheran Mission	49,956	1	6
Church Missionary Society	93,873	–	–
UMCA (Masasi Diocese)	26,344	2 main 3 small	2
UMCA (Zanzibar Diocese)	160,927	7 2 maternity	10[†]

Notes
* Mission figures taken from summaries of medical mission work provided to Medical Department; Church Missionary Society: TNA 450 692 v.1 'Medical Work in the Diocese of Central Tanganyika', to Medical Department, 13 October 1936; UMCA, 'The Medical Work of the UMCA in Masasi Diocese. The returns cover statistics from 1935, or the year to mid-1936. Government figures taken from Government of Tanzania, *Annual Report of the Medical Department, 1945*, Dar es Salaam: Government printer, 1947, p. 24
† In addition to its 10 dispensaries, the UMCA had 8 'district dispensaries' for which figures for out-patients have not been provided. In 1936 government medical services treated 598,016 out-patients.

focused on key areas of welfare delivery – especially education and health, where constraints and opportunities were similar for the majority of missions – and did not seek to broaden its ecumenical approach to matters theological or spiritual. Efforts to create umbrella organisations for coordinating mission activity at the international level in the post-war period were, perhaps inevitably, more controversial, especially within the Protestant faith. The World Council of Churches (WCC), in its broadly (and inevitably, given the range of churches it sought accommodate) ecumenical approach was regarded by some on the more evangelical wing with suspicion, or even outright disdain. W.O.H. Garman, President of the American Council of Christian Churches (ACCC), denounced the emergence of the WCC as one of the 'forces of anti-Christ' for its attempt 'to gain a totalitarian and monopolistic control of the missionary situation throughout the world'.[26] John Mackay, President of the International Missionary Council, was attacked by Garman for his alleged links to 'communist-front organisations' and his presence at a meeting where delegates 'prayed to the Virgin Mary, a host of saints, and for the dead'.[27] Yet within Tanganyika, organisations which would refuse to join the WCC on religious grounds neverthe-less worked with organisations such as the TMC which functioned in similar ways to the WCC, albeit at the national level. The Africa Inland Mission, for example, was a member of the Christian Council of Tanganyika, whilst remaining (in the early 1950s at least) wary of the WCC. Indeed, Reverend Maynard, the long-standing missionary at Kola Ndoto (and whose wife had been one of Tanganyika's most influential and significant mission doctors), wrote to the General-Secretary of the Africa Inland Mission (AIM) criticising views such as Garman's as not only being wrong but potentially undermining mission activity in East Africa.[28]

In bringing together mission medical practitioners from different (Protestant) churches to formulate common positions, the MMC (and from 1952 the ecumenical MMAC) created in the mission medical sphere an identity that transcended (but did not replace) individual mission identities, just as the TMC did for broader (Protestant) mission identity. In sharing experiences and problems, mission doctors and nurses identified cross-denominational constraints, challenges, opportunities and potential threats. The existence of the MMC served to entrench the picture of a sector meeting the health needs of Africans. A single mission might have few hospital beds or practitioners. But working alongside their co-religionists under the MMC, they formed a health sector that rivalled that of the state in its reach. For medical missionary work, it was perhaps less the chance to work with government than the potential to challenge its policies as they affected medical mission services that presented the real opportunity for a new faith sector to flex its muscles and demonstrate its strength through unity.

'Political implications': cooperation and competition between the MMC and the colonial state

If the primary impetus for the establishment of the TMC and MMC as the voice of the mission sector came from mission leaders themselves, the colonial administration was broadly supportive of these efforts, seeing in them an initiative that could enhance government–mission relations.[29] However, whilst recognising the possibilities for more coordinated efforts, and for a more effective utilisation of mission capacity, it was reluctant to see the TMC evolve into an organisation with real power over the policy-making process. Missions could inform government of their views, but were to be excluded from access to influence:

Government's present concern was mainly with the educational work of the various missions and the need for its coordination with the State enterprise. The Educational Advisory Committee should achieve this purpose provided it was properly and authoritatively informed of the views of the missionary organisations.[30]

For the government, the principal benefit of the TMC was to formulate a coherent mission sector voice, enabling the government to work with a single organisation rather than face the cumbersome task of dealing with each individual missionary society in turn. Moreover, it saw the main area of engagement as the education sector, rather than the medical one. Missions were to be neither encouraged nor expected to take on a more proactive role in shaping colonial policy in the social services.

Meetings of the MMC, attended by the Director of Medical Services (DMS) and other medical officers, were opportunities to press for changes to policy, clarification and support. Greater cooperation and coordination with government was seen as an important area. At a meeting in September 1937 the MMC requested that government inform missions of its plans for constructing hospitals and dispensaries, in order to avoid 'overlapping in work which resulted in wasted effort and in some cases financial losses to Missions'. The meeting also offered advice to the DMS on what the MMC perceived as failures in Medical Department policy. The practice of using unmarried young women as midwives, it advised, was counterproductive, and mission practices of using older, married mothers were more culturally acceptable. The perennial question of the relationship with Native Authority health services was addressed, in this instance whether mission medical practitioners had the right to step in when they noted bad practice (the answer was 'no'). The MMC asked the DMS to permit nurses to handle limited quantities of 'dangerous drugs' where no physician was resident (agreed, subject to notification to government). The DMS also agreed to raise the question of rail freight charges for essential medicines and medical equipment with the railways (although he did not have the power himself to enforce changes in policy).[31] The following year, at a meeting between missionary representatives (including Catholic) and the Medical Department, the agenda covered methylated spirit regulations; fees charged by mission dispensaries; rail freight charges; dental practice; leprosy control; and efforts against hookworm.[32] Whilst such meetings allowed missions to raise concerns, the government seemed to view them more as information-gathering sessions than as opportunities to seriously change policies in the light of mission recommendations. Nevertheless, the colonial medical department was keen to find solutions and compromises where possible. The meeting of 1937, for example, requested a change in the law to allow mission dispensers and dressers to charge fees without breaking the law: such fees were to the mission, not the individual, and were payments for drugs and dressings administered, not consultation or advice (which was free of charge). The DMS was adamant that the law could not be amended. However, he remained 'sympathetic towards the charging of fees where it is made quite clear that proper attention is being given for free'.[33] In respect of high freight charges for drugs and equipment, the DMS advised missions to forward him details of discrepancies and high charges for particular items, promising that he would liaise with the railways department. The DMS also agreed to inform the MMC of government plans to open or close dispensaries, in order to better coordinate with mission provision.[34]

Where missions had a particularly dominant role to play, such as in the treatment and care for leprosy sufferers, government was even more careful to involve the MMC in an advisory capacity. Following the publication of a report on Tanganyika's leprosy services, missions 'will be given opportunity for discussion of these recommendations and consultation with Government', the Chief Secretary assured the MMC in 1948.[35] As part of the 1952 review of government policy towards medical mission, the MMC was asked for 'suggestions' as to future cooperation.[36]

If 'cooperation' was the potential gain to be made from working with a single mission representative organisation, maintaining exclusive control over policy discussion and formulation became, inevitably, the chief site of conflict between TMC/MMC and the colonial state. Whilst it welcomed the desire of missions to work more closely with it, the Tanganyikan administration remained cautious of moving too far in formalising such a role. 'The Government appreciates the importance of securing the widest cooperation of all who are interested in the ... social services', the Chief Secretary wrote in 1944 in a letter to the Secretary of the TMC, 'and will gladly avail itself of opportunities for suggesting such participation as they arise.'[37] But such cooperation was to remain *ad hoc*, with a barely disguised resistance to any formalisation of procedures:

> The Government has taken full note of the recommendation made that wherever practicable and possible the Missions should be allowed to take part in planning social services developments in the Territory, and hopes to be able to act upon it from time to time as suitable occasions arise.[38]

But such caution increasingly cut across the realities of the critical role played by missions in healthcare provision. By 1950, the Medical Department had agreed that the MMC should be formally recognised by the department, which should also attend MMC committee meetings to 'discuss matters of common interest'.[39] Notably, despite this, no formal invitation was extended at this moment to the MMC to attend, as an official member, discussions within the Medical Department.

By 1948, however, the colonial administration had already ceded a major concession to the missions in the form of extending grants-in-aid for mission services from education to the medical sector. Until the late 1930s, the government made no regular payments for mission medical services. Missions applied each year, with no guarantee of future commitment, for the limited money paid out by the state to voluntary sector health services. In 1936, the colonial state made relatively small grants totalling £4,309 (out of a total budget of £185,735) to medical missions: £1,644 for the maintenance of leprosy camps; £1,356 for Lutindi Mental Hospital, run by the UMCA; £971 for mission maternal and child health services; £319 for drugs (including drugs for leprosy treatment); and £19 to cover mission assistance in 'epidemic outbreaks'.[40] Fearing that 'the grant of assistance directly from [government] funds to one mission is likely to lead to demands from others', the state avoided creating what it felt would result in a 'more or less unlimited obligation' by refusing to move to a formal grants-in-aid policy as it had done for education.[41] Indeed, the government feared that one major motivation behind the establishment of the MMC was precisely to lobby for such an obligation. The push towards 'closer cooperation between medical missionaries and the medical department', the DMS noted in 1937, was 'largely a financial question'. Moreover, the DMS noted, there were also 'political implications'.[42] The MMC was seeking not only to increase government financial commitments to mission facilities but also to 'make recommendations as to grants'.[43]

Despite government reluctance to countenance such a development, the increased presence of missionary medical services as a distinct sector, better highlighting the contribution made by missions to health-care in Tanganyika, made the move towards grants-in-aid for medical missions increasingly difficult to resist. As early as 1933 the government had conceded its willingness to 'consider sympathetically applications for assistance in special lines of work having a direct bearing on public health, such as maternity and child welfare, anti-venereal diseases, and yaws work, leprosy and hookworm and the like'.[44] Four years later, the DMS suggested that in places where there was no colonial medical officer, '[f]ormal agreements might be entered into and scales of remuneration laid down' where missions agreed to undertake work that would otherwise have been done by a state physician.[45]

Given this history of increasing agitation for closer formal ties, it is not surprising that the plans for post-war medical development in 1943 recognised the mission sector as playing a critical role:

> to the extent that medical missionary effort may comply with such standards as may be determined from the standards set for the Government and Native Authority medical services, as well as the training of medical and nursing auxiliaries and other trained subordinates; to that extent such effort should be state-aided.[46]

In return for greater regulation of mission medical services, and commitments that such services would treat all, regardless of faith (and in effect become a core part of the embryonic national health system), it was agreed that missions would receive regular grants-in-aid in support of their work. The proposals were formalised in the Medical (Grants-in-Aid to Missions) Regulations of 1948, and the Medical (Training Grants-in-Aid to Missions) Regulations that were published the following year in Tanganyika. In 1956, some twenty years after missions had shared a £4,309 state contribution to their efforts, grants-in-aid to mission medical services (including payments for staff, hospitals and training) amounted to £101,013.[47]

If having ceded the principle of direct government funding for mission services left the state, by the end of the 1940s, believing that it had gone far enough in accommodating mission demands, the question of influence was not yet finished for the MMC/MMAC. Tensions over exactly how much power medical mission should have in framing colonial medical policy were brought to a head in the discussions over the creation of the MMAC in 1952. The MMC presented a robust conception of the role the new organisation ought to play in relation to medical policy within Tanganyika, seeing the institution's remit as being 'to assist in administration of the Grant in Aid regulations, and to advise the Director of Medical Services on all matters related to or affecting the medical work of Missions in the Territory'.[48] For the administration, this was presumptuous. The idea that 'regulations, as approved by Executive Council, should be referred back to this Committee for *their* further consideration', B. Leechman, the member for social services wrote, 'is out of the question'.[49] The government was determined that power should remain within the Medical Department alone. 'While it is to be expected that you will most certainly consult this Advisory Committee', Leechman wrote to the DMS, 'I think it most desirable to do nothing to suggest that there is an obligation upon you to seek advice or, most particularly, that it is necessary to act in accordance with that advice.'[50] The DMS similarly regarded such a committee as a challenge to the authority of the government to direct grants-in-aid policy without reference to other actors, writing:

I do not quite understand what Miss Phillips means when she asks that the Committee should be set up early in order to discuss the future administration of grants-in-aid. If she means merely to discuss the administration of these grants within the framework of the Regulations which have been passed on the Executive Council's agreed policy, then I have no objection; but if she wishes at this juncture to have a meeting to discuss change of policy, I do not think there is much to be gained in doing so.[51]

However, while the higher echelons of the colonial administration were appalled by the idea of granting such privileged access to voluntary non-state actors, the Medical Department itself was more realistic about the need for a flexible approach. The DMS agreed that the new advisory body should be 'consultative', stating that whilst 'ultimate discretion lies with the Director of Medical Services',[52] he nevertheless recognised the importance of maintaining good links with the mission sector. 'I anticipate needless trouble if all reference is excluded [to such a mission role], and I would deprecate any step likely to affect adversely our relationships with the missions which I should say are probably better today than they have ever been.'[53]

In the event, the MMAC was established to 'advise the Director of Medical Services on all matters relating to or affecting the medical work of Missions in the Territory'.[54] Its remit echoed almost exactly the terms suggested by the Secretary of the MMC. It consisted of four state representatives, including the DMS, and four mission representatives, appointed by the MMC. The state could not reject the logic that it had helped to create. If missions were a constituent element of a national health system – a system that the missions had helped to create through their negotiations and interactions with the state through the MMC in particular – then their influence could not be ignored. By coming together, diluting the strength of the individual, missions had created a sector that could wield significant power through collective action and identity. The colonial state was not beholden to, or subjugated by, missions in the medical sphere. Indeed, missions had themselves entered a state of increased dependence upon the state as a consequence of their increased access to and influence in the Medical Department. And that mutual dependence also characterised the emergent health system: dependent upon two distinct partners working together, each helping to counteract the weaknesses of the other, and based upon actors who, ultimately, were outsiders and subject to power dynamics in the communities in which they operated, which meant they could never truly claim to be sanctioned by or reflect local demands, needs and wants.

Conclusion

The health system created by the partnership of colonial state and mission providers, the mix of public and private (voluntary) provision, would last until the nationalisations of the 1970s,[55] and then re-emerge from the late 1980s onwards, when many churches were given back control over the medical facilities they had once operated as missions. At the moment of independence, missions contributed hugely to the official welfare services provided for directly and indirectly by the colonial state. In 1961, missions provided 8,350 beds in hospitals and clinics, compared to just over 7,000 under the direct control of the Medical Department. In that year missions treated 152,298 in-patients, and over 4.5 million out-patients. Government services treated only slightly more: 160,941 in-patients and 4.9 million out-patients. Six years later, at the time of the publication of the Arusha Declaration and the formal adoption of Ujamaa, missions still had over 11,000 beds and were treating 6.3 million out-patients (compared to the state's 7,890 beds and 9.9 million out-patients).[56] As this chapter has sought to demonstrate, 'colonial medicine' in Tanganyika was varied, complex and functioned as a public-private partnership in which missions were formal, recognised partners in the delivery of healthcare to Africans across the territory. However, the construction of this model of health-care delivery required missions to conceptualise themselves as belonging to a clearly designated 'sector'. From the mid-1930s, in partnership with the colonial state, which saw the advantages of cooperating with missions as an organised collective rather than atomised individuals, missions constructed institutions which would bind them together in facing the state.

In terms of the health sector, this set in train the slow formalisation of a partnership between the state and the voluntary (mission) sector that extended government regulation over mission facilities, but at the same time gave mission representatives a greater and more powerful voice within the administration. Mission hospitals and clinics had dominated healthcare in the rural areas since the late nineteenth century. With the establishment of the TMC and MMC, the engagement with the Medical Department that followed and the gradual extension of grants-in-aid to medical mission, they were transformed into a formal, albeit distinct, part of colonial health service provision in Tanganyika. This story has importance beyond what it tells us about colonial medicine, however. Looking beyond the importance of constructing a fuller narrative of the multifaceted constitution of 'colonial medicine' in Tanganyika, the emergence of the mission sector as a non-state voluntary provider of welfare services also has implications for post-colonial history. Firstly, it raises questions about analyses that see the period of the 1980s as critical in shifting from a public to private sector model of service delivery (in particular, as much of the literature suggests, based upon the non-governmental organisation (NGO)). The story of national ownership of public services in Tanzania is a complex one but, in the sense of full nationalisation, it is also a short one. Effectively by the 1930s, and formally with the passing of the 1948 Medical (Grants-in-Aid to Missions) Regulation, healthcare services in Tanganyika were a public-private hybrid: largely funded by the state, provided by a partnership between public and voluntary actors. The encroachment of NGOs into the public space from the 1980s was, then, not something new, but a recasting of older forms of delivery of public goods. It rested upon a different set of ideological foundations, but was based within and upon a voluntary sector space that had been created in the colonial period.

Secondly, the establishment of a 'mission sector' in welfare provision and development intervention leads us to question accounts of the 'voluntary sector' that exclude, marginalise or completely ignore missions. As this chapter has shown, missions were not just part of the creation of this sector, but its originators and first actors. The development of the sector since independence (in which faith-based organisations have continued to play a major part) has evolved in new ways and in response to newly emerging impulses. But the sets of relationships with the state, with informal voluntary actors (those which have not been officially recognised and drawn into formal channels and structures), with international actors and with the communities in which they undertake interventions, were first cast and subsequently shaped by missions in the colonial period. Any account and history of voluntary action in sub-Saharan Africa must recognise this.

Finally, the chapter has asked questions of how we understand colonial welfare policies and services. The easy assumption that welfare was simply a con, softening the hard blow of colonial occupation, becomes harder to maintain when one looks to the diversity of actors engaged in welfare provision. Missions were never simply agents of Empire, and their relationship with imperial aims varies between missions and individual missionaries, and across time and place, to create a highly complex set of interactions and relations. That is not to deny the cynical opportunism, economic strategic thinking and highly unequal power relationships and racialised stereotypes that underlay much of colonial welfare. But we cannot assume that what drove the Medical Department in, say, early 1950s Tanganyika was reflected in the views espoused by all missions engaged and employed by that state. Much has been written on the provision of public goods in post-colonial Africa.

[170]

Those debates also need to be had for the colonial period, allowing for a grander narrative of welfare service provision in Africa that transcends colonial boundaries and considers all influences and impulses that created and shaped welfare and social development.

Notes

1   R.M. Titmuss, *The Health Services of Tanganyika: A Report to the Government*, London, Pitman Medical Publishing Co., 1964, p. 1
2   M. Turshen, 'The Impact of Colonialism on Health and Health Services in Tanzania', *International Journal of Health Services*, 7, 1977, pp. 7–35
3   T. Ranger, 'Godly Medicine: The Ambiguities of Medical Mission in Southeastern Tanzania, 1900–1945', in S. Feierman and John M Janzen (eds.), *The Social Basis of Health and Healing in Africa*, Berkeley, University of California Press, 1992, p. 257
4   David Hardiman, 'Introduction', in David Hardiman (ed.), *Healing Bodies, Saving Souls: Medical Missions in Asia and Africa*, Amsterdam and New York, Rodopi, 2006, p. 20
5   Ana Madeira, 'Portuguese, French and British Discourses on Colonial Education: Church–State Relations, School Expansion and Missionary Competition in Africa, 1890–1930', *Paedagogica Historica*, 41, 1/2, 2005, p. 38
6   Colonial claims on this can, however, be contested. See Michael Jennings, '"Healing of Bodies, Salvation of Souls"': Missionary Medicine in Colonial Tanganyika, 1870s–1939', *Journal of Religion in Africa*, 38, 2008, pp. 27–56
7   Tanzania National Archive (TanNA) 450 692. V. 1 Church Missionary Society, 'Medical Work in the Diocese of Central Tanganyika', report to Medical Department, 13 October 1936
8   Michael Jennings, '"A Matter of Vital Importance": The Place of Medical Mission in Maternal and Child Healthcare in Tanganyika, 1919–39', in David Hardiman (ed.), *Medical Missionaries in India and Africa*, Amsterdam and New York, Rodopi, 2006, pp. 227–50
9   TanNA File 712 Shinyanga District Annual Report 1926, pp. 29–30
10 TanNA File 712 Shinyanga District Annual Report 1926, p. 30
11 TanNA File 712 Shinyanga District Annual Report 1931, p. 37. Although a Native Authority institution, the maternity home had been set up and was run by Dr Maynard. It therefore functioned in effect as a mission medical service. For more details about the Africa Inland Mission's maternity clinic, see Jennings, 'Missions and Maternal and Child Health Care'.
12 TanNA 450 692 v.1 UMCA, 'The Medical Work of the UMCA in Masasi Diocese'
13 Tanganyika Government, *Report on Health Services 1959: vol. II (Statistics and Technical Papers)*, Dar es Salaam, Government Printer, 1960, pp. 15–16, 21. Around 1.7 per cent of out-patients in government facilities were Asian or European.
14 Edwin W. Smith, *The Christian Mission in Africa: A Study Based on the Proceedings of the International Conference at Le Zoute, Belgium, September 14th to 21st, 1926*, London, International Missionary Council, 1926, p. 120–1
15 TanNA 21247, v.1 Bishop of Masasi, Letter to Missions, 5 November 1937
16 TanNA 21247, v.1 Bishop of Masasi, Letter to Missions, 5 November 1937
17 TanNA 21247 v.1 Chief Secretary (?) note of interview, 24 December 1932
18 Michael Jennings, 'Common Counsel, Common Policy: Healthcare, Missions and the Rise of the "Voluntary Sector" in Colonial Tanzania', *Development and Change*, 44, 4, 2013, pp. 939–63
19 TanNA 21247 v.2 TMC Minutes, 12–14 May 1948
20 TanNA 24848 Director of Medical Services to the Chief Secretary, 25 February 1937
21 TanNA 450 692 v.1 Secretary Berliner Mission to Director of Medical Services, 6 July 1936
22 TanNA 450 692 v.1 Muller, 'Medical Mission and its Relations to Government'; the

document is undated and no author is mentioned, but it is the paper mentioned in the agenda of the TMC meeting, 9–11 July 1936 (TanNA 21247 v.1), where Dr Muller is named as the author.

23 TanNA 450 692 v.1 Director of Medical Services to Chief Secretary, February 1937
24 TanNA 10721 v.5 Constitution of the Medical Missionary Committee, 1951
25 TanNA 42293 Director of Medical Services to Medical Missionary Committee (1283/1/467), cited in Minutes of Meeting of Mission Medical Committee, 22–23 January 1952. Whilst the CCT remained interested and engaged in mission-provided social services, and relations with the colonial state over their provision, it represented its Protestant members, rather than adopting an ecumenical approach.
26 TanNA 12586, v.2 W.O.H. Garman, President ACCC, 'Foreign Missions Crisis', *The Voice*, December 1949, p. 8
27 TanNA 12586, v.2 W.O.H. Garman, President ACCC, 'Foreign Missions Crisis', *The Voice*, December 1949, p. 8
28 TanNA 12586, v.2 Rev. Maynard to Rev. R.T. Davis, General-Secretary African Inland Mission, 20 March 1950. Interestingly, in describing the CCT, Maynard was keen to stress 'the [CCT] is a local organisation having no official connection with any other organisation outside itself, not even with the [Christian Council of Kenya]'.
29 TanNA 21247, v.1 Chief Secretary to Governor (?), 16 December 1932
30 TanNA 21247 v.1 Chief Secretary (?) note of interview, 24 December 1932
31 TanNA 450 692 v.1 Minutes of the Meeting of the Medical Committee of the Tanganyika Missionary Council, 16 September 1937
32 TanNA 24848, UMCA to MMC Members, 18 June 1938
33 TanNA 450 692 v.1 Minutes of the Meeting of the Medical Committee of the Tanganyika Missionary Council, 16 September 1937
34 TanNA 24848 Director of Medical Services to Chief Secretary, 14 October 1937, p. 2
35 TanNA 21247 v.2 Tanganyika Missionary Council Minutes, 12–14 May 1948
36 TanNA 42293 Miss Phillips (Secretary MMC) to Member for Social Services, 29 July 1952
37 TanNA 21247 v.2 Chief Secretary (G.R. Sandford), to Secretary, Tanganyika Missionary Council (Rev. Canon R. Banks, Church Missionary Society Kilimatinde), 14 September 1944
38 TanNA 21247 v.2 Chief Secretary (G.R. Sandford), to Secretary, Tanganyika Missionary Council (Rev. Canon R. Banks, Church Missionary Society Kilimatinde), 14 September 1944
39 TanNA 42300 Minutes of meeting of Medical Grants-in-Aid Committee, 12 January 1950
40 TanNA 450 692 v.1 Government grants to missions for 1936 taken from Director of Medical Services to Chief Secretary, 10 August 1937; government expenditure for 1936 taken from Government of Tanganyika, *Annual Report of the Medical Department, 1945*, Dar es Salaam: Government Printer, 1947, p. 24
41 TanNA 10721 v.1 Secretariat Minutes, 27 June 1927; 17 November 1927
42 TanNA 24848 Secretariat Minutes, Director of Medical Services, 25 August 1937
43 TanNA 24848 Secretariat Minutes, 27 February 1937
44 TanNA AN450 178/3 Secretariat Minute, Director of Medical and Sanitary Services, 4 December 1933
45 TanNA 24843 Director of Medical Services, Cooperation with Missions, memorandum, 1937
46 TanNA AN 450 1179 Director of Medical Services (P.A.T. Sneath), 'Post-War Development – Medical Department', September 1943, pp. 2–3
47 Government of Tanganyika, *Annual Report of the Medical Department 1956*, Dar es Salaam, Government Printer, 1957, p. 37
48 TanNA 42300 Miss Phillips, Medical Missionary Council, to Director of Medical Services, 13 August 1952
49 TanNA 42300 B. Leechman, Member for Social Services, to Director of Medical Services, 26 September 1952 (emphasis in the original)

50 TanNA 42300 B. Leechman, Member for Social Services, to Director of Medical Services, 26 September 1952
51 TanNA 42300 Director of Medical Services to Member for Social Services, 16 September 1952
52 TanNA 42300 Director of Medical Services to Member for Social Services (B. Leechman), 15 November 1952
53 TanNA 42300 Director of Medical Services to Member for Social Services (B. Leechman), 15 November 1952
54 TanNA 42300 *Tanganyika Gazette*, 19 December 1952
55 Nationalisation of the health system never amounted to much more than the government taking over a few mission hospitals, many of which were soon returned to their original owners.
56 Tanganyika Government, *Medical Department Annual Report, 1961*, vol. II, Dar es Salaam, Government Printer, 1962, and *Medical Department Annual Report, 1967*, vol. II, Dar es Salaam, Government Printer, 1968

BIBLIOGRAPHY

Primary sources

Archives and manuscripts

Africana manuscripts
British Empire manuscripts
British Library, London
British Medical Association Archive
Colonial Office papers
Dominions Committee Documents
East Africana Collection, Cory manuscripts
Furse papers
Government publications relating to Kenya, 1897–1963 (microfilm)
India Office Records
J.N.P. Davies papers
Kabale District Archives
Kenya National Archive records (microfilm)
Livingstonia Mission records
Malawi National Archives
Mwanza Archives
National Archives of Ghana, Accra
National Library of Scotland
Nigerian National Archives, Ibadan
Papers of Winifred Annie Milnes-Walker
Rhodes House Library, Oxford
Twohig papers
Syracuse University
Tanzania National Archives
The National Archives, Kew (UK)
University of Birmingham Special Collections
Uganda Mission records
University of Dar es Salaam
Women's Library, London
Zanzibar National Archives

Printed sources

Anon, 'Asiatics Salaries Cut: Indian Reply to Geddes Committee Suggestion', *The Leader*, 20 May 1922, p. 8
Anon, 'Mass Meeting and Dr Burkitt', *East African Chronicle*, 13 August 1921
Colonial Office, *Miscellaneous No. 488: The Colonial Service, General Conditions of Employment*, London, The Colonial Office, 1939

Colonial Office, 'Report of the Committee Chaired by Sir Warren Fisher', *The System of Appointment in the Colonial Office and the Colonial Services*, London, HMSO, 1930

Colonial Office, *Miscellaneous No. 99: Colonial Medical Appointments*, London, The Colonial Office, 1921

Colonial Office, Cmd. 939 *Report of the Departmental Committee Appointed by the Secretary of State for the Colonies to Enquire into the Colonial Medical Services*, London, HMSO, 1920

East African Medical Survey, *Annual Report, 1953*, Nairobi, EAHC, 1954

East African Medical Survey, *Annual Report, 1952*, Nairobi EAHC, 1953

Free Church of Scotland Monthly Record, January 1901

Government of Kenya, 'An Ordinance to make Provision for the Registration of Medical Practitioners and Dentists through the 1910 Medical Practitioners and Dentists Ordinance', *The Official Gazette*, 1 October 1910

Government of Tanganyika, *Annual Report of the Medical Department 1956*, Dar es Salaam, Government Printer, 1957

Government of Tanganyika, *Annual Report of the Medical Department, 1945*, Dar es Salaam: Government Printer, 1947

Kenya Colony, Public Health Ordinance, Nairobi, Kenya, Government Printers, 1921

Laurie, W. and H. Trant, *East African Medical Survey, Monograph no. 2: A Health Survey in Bukoba District, Tanganyika*, Nairobi, EAHC, 1954

Livingstonia Mission, *Annual Report of the Livingstonia Mission for 1910*, Glasgow, 1911

Nyasaland Protectorate, *Annual Medical Report for 1930*, Zomba, 1931

Nyasaland Protectorate, *Annual Medical Report for 1928*, Zomba, 1929

Nyasaland Protectorate, *Annual Medical Report for 1924*, Zomba, 1925

Nyasaland Protectorate, *Annual Medical Report for 1914*, Zomba, 1915

Nyasaland Protectorate, *Report of Commissioner for 1912–1913*, Cmd. 7050, London, 1913

Simpson, W.J., *Report on the Sanitary Matters in the East Africa Protectorate, Uganda and Zanzibar*, London, Colonial Office, Africa No. 1025, February 1915

Tanganyika Government, *Medical Department Annual Report, 1967*, vol. II, Dar es Salaam, Government Printer, 1968

Tanganyika Government, *Medical Department Annual Report, 1961*, vol. II, Dar es Salaam, Government Printer, 1962

Tanganyika Government, *Report on Health Services 1959: vol. II (Statistics and Technical Papers)*, Dar es Salaam, Government Printer, 1960

Tanganyika Territory, *Annual Report of the Medical Department 1943*, Dar es Salaam, Government Printer, 1944

Tanganyika Territory, *Annual Report of the Medical Department 1941*, Dar es Salaam, Government Printer, 1942

Tanganyika Territory, *Annual Medical report 1938*, Dar es Salaam, Government Printer, 1940

[175]

Tanganyika Territory, *Department of Agriculture Annual Report, 1932*, Dar es Salaam: Government Printer, 1933

The Livingstonia News, October 1909

Uganda Protectorate, *Annual Medical Report, 1952*, Entebbe, Government Printer, 1953

Uganda Protectorate, *Annual Medical and Sanitary Report for the Year Ended 31st December, 1925*, Entebbe, Government Printer, Uganda, 1926

Uganda Protectorate, *Annual Medical and Sanitary Report for the Year Ended 31st December, 1919*, Entebbe, Government Printer, Uganda, 1920

Welbourn, H., *Our Children*, Kampala, Uganda Council of Women, n.d. [c.1960]

Zanzibar Protectorate, *Annual Medical Report, 1937*, Zanzibar, Government Printer, 1938

Zanzibar Protectorate, *Annual Medical Report, 1934*, Zanzibar, Government Printer, 1935

Zanzibar Protectorate, *Annual Medical Report, 1933*, Zanzibar, Government Printer, 1934

Zanzibar Protectorate, *Annual Medical Report, 1932*, Zanzibar, Government Printer, 1933

Zanzibar Protectorate, *Annual Medical Report, 1930*, Zanzibar, Government Printer, 1931

Zanzibar Protectorate, *Annual Medical Report, 1928*, Zanzibar, Government Printer, 1929

Zanzibar Protectorate, *Annual Medical Report, 1927*, Zanzibar, Government Printer, 1928

Zanzibar Protectorate, *Annual Medical Report, 1925*, Zanzibar, Government Printer, 1926

Zanzibar Protectorate, *Annual Medical Report, 1924*, Zanzibar, Government Printer, 1925

Zanzibar Protectorate, *Annual Medical Report, 1923*, Zanzibar, Government Printer, 1924

Zanzibar Protectorate, *Annual Medical Report, 1922*, Zanzibar, Government Printer, 1923

Zanzibar Protectorate, *Annual Medical Report, 1921*, Zanzibar, Government Printer, 1922

Zanzibar Protectorate, *Annual Medical Report, 1918*, Zanzibar, Government Printer, 1919

Secondary works

Adeloye, Adeloya, *African Pioneers of Modern Medicine: Nigerian Doctors of the Nineteenth Century*, Ibadan, University Press Limited, 1985

Ainsworth, M., *Infancy in Uganda: Infant Care and the Growth of Love*, Baltimore, Johns Hopkins Press, 1967

Aiyar, Sana, 'Empire, Race and the Indians in Colonial Kenya's Contested Public Political Sphere, 1919–1923', *Africa: The Journal of the International African Institute*, 81, 1, 2011, pp. 132–54

Allen, Denise Roth, *Managing Motherhood, Managing Risk: Fertility and Danger in West Central Tanzania*, Ann Arbor, The University of Michigan Press, 2002

Anderson, David, *Histories of the Hanged: The Dirty War in Kenya and the End of Empire*, London, Weidenfeld and Nicolson, 2005

Anderson, Warwick, *Colonial Pathologies: American Tropical Medicine, Race and Hygiene in the Philippines*, Durham, NC, Duke University Press, 2006

Anderson, Warwick, 'Excremental Colonialism: Public Health and the Poetics of Pollution', *Critical Enquiry*, 21, 1995, pp. 640–69

Anderson, W., D. Jenson and R. Keller (eds.), *Unconscious Dominions: Psychoanalysis, Colonial Trauma, and Global Sovereignties*, Durham, NC, Duke University Press, 2011

Anon, 'Meetings of Branches and Divisions', *Supplement to the British Medical Journal*, 11 July 1936, p. 29

Anon, 'Asiatics Salaries Cut: Indian Reply to Geddes Committee Suggestion', *The Leader*, 20 May 1922

Anon, 'Mass Meeting and Dr Burkitt', *East African Chronicle*, 13 August 1921

Anon, 'Instruction in Tropical Diseases', *British Medical Journal*, i, 1895, p. 771

Arnold, David, *Science, Technology and Medicine in Colonial India*, Cambridge, Cambridge University Press, 2000

Arnold, David, *Colonizing the Body: State Medicine and Epidemic Disease in Nineteenth Century India*, Berkeley, University of California Press, 1993

Attewell, Guy, *Refiguring Unani Tibb: Plural Healing in Late Colonial India*, Hyderabad, India, Orient Longman, 2007

Austen, R., *Northwest Tanzania under German and British Rule: Colonial Policy and Tribal Politics, 1889-1939*, New Haven, Yale University Press, 1968

Baker, Colin, 'The Government Medical Service in Malawi: an Administrative History, 1891–1974', *Medical History*, 20, 1976, pp. 296–311

Baker, Colin, 'The Development of the Administration to 1897', in Bridglal Pachai (ed.), *The Early History of Malawi*, London, Northwestern University Press, 1972, pp. 323–43

Bala, Poonam, *Imperialism and Medicine in Bengal*, New Delhi, Sage Publications, 1991

Balfour, Andrew and Henry Harold Scott, *Health Problems of the Empire: Past, Present and Future*, London, W. Collins Sons and Co., Ltd., 1924

Barber, Charles, *Comfortably Numb: How Psychiatry Is Medicating a Nation*, New York, Pantheon Books, 2008

Bayoumi, A., *The History of the Sudan Health Services*, Nairobi, Kenya Literature Bureau, 1979

Beck, Ann, *A History of the British Medical Administration of East Africa: 1900–1950*, Cambridge, MA, Harvard University Press, 1970

Beidelman, T., *Colonial Evangelism: A Socio-Historical Study of an East African Mission at the Grassroots*, Bloomington IN, Indiana University Press, 1982

Bell, Heather, *Frontiers of Medicine in the Anglo-Egyptian Sudan, 1899–1940*, Oxford, Clarendon Press 1999

Bell, Leland V., *Mental and Social Disorder in Sub-Saharan Africa: The Case of Sierra Leone, 1787–1990*, Westport, CT, Greenwood Press, 1991

Bennett, Brett M. and Joseph M. Hodge (eds.), *Science and Empire: Knowledge and Networks of Science across the British Empire, 1800–1970*, Basingstoke, Palgrave Macmillan, 2011

Berman, Bruce and John Lonsdale, *Unhappy Valley: Conflict in Kenya and Africa [Book 1 State and Class]*, London, James Currey, 1991

Bhacker, M. Reda, *Trade and Empire in Muscat and Zanzibar: the Roots of British Domination*, London, Routledge, 1992

Bharati, Agehananda, *The Asians in East Africa: Jayhind and Uhuru*, Chicago, Nelson-Hall Co., 1972

Bhattacharya, Sanjoy with Sharon Messenger, *The Global Eradication of Smallpox*, Hyderabad, Orient Black Swan, 2010

Bhattacharya, Sanjoy, *Expunging Variola: The Control and Eradication of Smallpox in India, 1947–1977*, New Delhi and London, Orient Longman India and Sangam Books, 2006

Bhattacharya, Sanjoy, Mark Harrison and Michael Worboys (eds.), *Fractured States: Smallpox, Public Health and Vaccination Policy in British India, 1800–1947*, New Delhi, Orient Longman and Sangam Books, 2005

Billington, W.R., 'Albert Cook: A Biographical Note', *East African Medical Journal*, 28, 1951, pp. 397–422

Blyth, Robert J., *The Empire of the Raj: India, Eastern Africa and the Middle East, 1858–1947*, Cambridge, Cambridge University Press, 2003

Bödeker, H.A., 'Some Sidelights on Early Medical History in East Africa', *The East African Medical Journal*, 12, 1935–36, pp. 100–7

Bowlby, J., *Maternal Care and Mental Health*, Geneva, 2nd edn, World Health Organization, Monograph Series, No. 2, 1952

Brantlinger, Patrick, 'Victorians and Africans: The Genealogy of the Myth of the Dark Continent.' *Critical Inquiry* 12, 1985, pp. 166–203

Bull, Mary, *The Medical Services of Tanganyika 1955*, Report 21, Oxford Development Records Project, Rhodes House Library, Oxford, [n.d. *c.*198?]

Bull, Mary, *The Medical Services of Uganda 1954–5*, Report 20, Oxford Development Records Project, Rhodes House Library, Oxford, [n.d. *c.*198?]

Burke-Gaffney, H.J.O.D., 'The History of Medicine in the African Countries', *Medical History*, 12, 1968, pp. 31–41

Calcutta Medical College, *The Centenary of the Medical College, Bengal, 1835–1934*, Calcutta, 1935

Carothers, J.C., *The African Mind in Health and Disease*, Geneva, World Health Organisation, 1955

Carothers, J., *The Psychology of Mau Mau*, Nairobi, Government Printer, 1954

Castellani, Aldo, *Microbes, Men and Monarchs: A Doctor's Life in Many Lands*, London, Gollancz, 1960

Chakrabarti, Pratik, *Medicine and Empire, 1600–1960*, London, Palgrave Macmillan, 2013

Chakrabarti, Pratik, *Western Science in Modern India: Metropolitan Methods, Colonial Practices*, Delhi, Permanent Black, 2004

Clyde, David F., *History of the Medical Services of Tanganyika*, Dar es Salaam, Government Press, 1962

Cobain, Ian, 'Revealed: the Bonfire of Papers at the End of Empire', *Guardian*, 29 November 2013

Cobain, Ian, 'Foreign Office Hoarding 1m Historic Files in Secret Archive', *Guardian*, 18 October 2013

Colonial Office, *Miscellaneous No. 488: The Colonial Service, General Conditions of Employment*, London, The Colonial Office, 1939

Colonial Office, 'Report of the Committee Chaired by Sir Warren Fisher', *The System of Appointment in the Colonial Office and the Colonial Services*, London, HMSO, 1930

Colonial Office, *Miscellaneous No. 99: Colonial Medical Appointments*, London, The Colonial Office, 1921

Colonial Office, Cmd. 939 *Report of the Departmental Committee Appointed by the Secretary of State for the Colonies to Enquire into the Colonial Medical Services*, London, HMSO, 1920

Comaroff, J., 'The Diseased Heart of Africa: Medicine, Colonialism, and the Black Body', in S. Lindenbaum and M. Lock (eds.), *Knowledge, Power, and Practice: the Anthropology of Medicine and Everyday Life*, Berkeley, California University Press, 1993, pp. 305–29

Cook, Albert Ruskin, *Uganda Memories, 1897–1940*, Kampala, Uganda Society, 1945

Cook, E.N., 'The Adventures of an X-Ray', *Mercy and Truth*, 276, 1920, pp. 277–81

Cook, E.N., 'A Medical Mission in War Time', *Mercy and Truth*, 216, 1914, pp. 392–4

Cook, J.H., 'A Year's Hospital Work in Central Africa', *Church Missionary Review*, 66, 1915, pp. 482–6

Cook, J.H., 'Missionaries and War Service', *Mercy and Truth*, 226, 1915, pp. 326–8

Cook, J.H., *9th Annual Report of Toro Medical Mission*, Torquay, C. Bendle, St. Mary Church Printing Works, 1911

Cook, J.H., 'Notes on Cases of "Sleeping Sickness" Occurring in the Uganda Protectorate', *Journal of Tropical Medicine*, 1901, p. 237

Cooper, F., *On the African Waterfront: Urban Disorder and the Transformation of Work in Colonial Mombasa*, New Haven, Yale University Press, 1987

Cordell, Dennis D., Joel W. Gregory and Victor Piché, *Hoe and Wage: A Social History of a Circular Migration System in West Africa*, Boulder, CO, Westview Press, 1996

Coupland, R., *East Africa and its Invaders From the Earliest Times to the Death of Seyyid Said*, London, Oxford University Press, 1938

Coupland, R., 'Zanzibar: an Asiatic Spice Island, Kirk and Slavery, *The Times*, 5 October 1928

Cox, Jeffrey, *Imperial Fault Lines: Christianity and Colonial Power in India, 1818–1940*, Stanford, CA, Stanford University Press, 2002

Cox, Jeffrey, 'Audience and Exclusion at the Margins of Imperial History', *Women's History Review*, 3, 4, 1994, pp. 501–14

Crofton, Richard Hayes, *Zanzibar Affairs*, 1914–1933, London, Francis Edwards, 1953

Crozier, Anna, 'What Was Tropical about Tropical Neurasthenia', *Journal of the History of Medicine and Allied Sciences*, 64, 2009, pp. 518–48

Crozier, Anna, *Practising Colonial Medicine: the Colonial Medical Service in British East Africa*, London, I.B. Tauris, 2007

Crozier, Anna, 'Sensationalising Africa: British Medical Impressions of Sub-Saharan Africa 1890–1939', *Journal of Imperial and Commonwealth History*, 35, 2007, pp. 393–415

Culwick, A. and G. Culwick, ed. V. Berry, *The Culwick Papers 1934–1944: Population, Food and Health in Colonial Tanganika*, London, Academic Books, 1994

Culwick, A. and G. Culwick, 'A Study of Population in Ulanga, Tanganyika Territory', *The Sociological Review*, 30, 1938, pp. 365–79

Curtin, P., 'Medical Knowledge and Urban Planning in Tropical Africa', *American Historical Review*, 90, 1985, pp. 594–613

Davies, J.N.P., 'The History of the Uganda Branch of the British Medical Association, 1913 to 1932', *East African Medical Journal*, 31, 1954, pp. 93–9

Davies, J., 'The Essential Pathology of Kwashiorkor', *The Lancet*, 1948, 1(6496), pp. 317–20

Davies, P.N., *The Trade Makers: Elder Dempster in West Africa, 1852–1972; 1973–1989*, St. John's, International Maritime Economic History Association, 2000

Davies, P.N., 'The Impact of the Expatriate Shipping Lines on the Economic Development of British West Africa', *Business History*, 19, 1977, pp. 3–17

Davin, Anna, 'Imperialism and Motherhood', in Frederick Cooper and Ann Laura Stoler (eds.), *Tensions of Empire: Colonial Cultures in a Bourgeois World*, Berkeley, University of California Press, 1997, pp. 87–151

Deacon, Harriet Jane, 'Madness, Race and Moral Treatment: Robben Island Lunatic Asylum, Cape Colony, 1846–1890', *History of Psychiatry*, vii, 1996, pp. 287–97

Delf, George, *Asians in East Africa*, Oxford University Press, 1963

Digby, Anne, 'The Mid-Level Health Worker in South Africa: The In-Between Condition of the "Middle"', in Ryan Johnson and Amna Khalid (eds.), *Public Health in the British Empire: Intermediaries, Subordinates, and the Practice of Public Health*, New York and London, Routledge, 2012, pp. 171–92

Digby, Anne, *Diversity and Division in Medicine: Healthcare in South Africa from the 1800s*, Oxford, Peter Lang, 2006

Digby, Anne, 'Early Black Doctors in South Africa', *Journal of African History*, 46, 2005, pp. 427–54

Digby, Anne and Helen Sweet, 'The Nurse as Culture Broker in Twentieth Century South Africa', in Waltraud Ernst (ed.), *Plural Medicine, Tradition and Modernity*, London, Routledge, 2002, pp. 113–29

Doyle, S., *Before HIV: Sexuality, Fertility and Mortality in East Africa, 1900–1980*, Oxford, Oxford University Press and the British Academy, 2013

Du Toit, B.M., *The Boers in East Africa: Ethnicity and Identity*, London, Bergen and Garvey, 1998

Ebrahimnejad, Hormoz (ed.), *The Development of Modern Medicine in Non-Western Countries: Historical Perspectives*, London and New York, Routledge, 2009

Ernst, Waltraud (ed.), *Plural Medicine, Tradition and Modernity*, London, Routledge, 2002

Fair, Laura, *Pastimes and Politics: Culture, Community, and Identity in Post-Abolition Urban Zanzibar, 1890–1945*, Athens, OH and London, Ohio University Press and James Currey, 2001

Fallers, L. (ed.), *All The King's Men: Leadership and Status in Buganda on the Eve of Independence*, London, Oxford University Press, 1964

Farley, John, *Bilharzia: A History of Imperial Tropical Medicine*, Cambridge, Cambridge University Press, 2008 [first published 1991]

Feierman, Steven, 'Struggles for Control: The Social Roots of Health and Healing in Modern Africa', *African Studies Review*, 28, 1985, pp. 73–147

Feierman, S. and J. Janzen (eds.), *The Social Basis of Health and Healing in Africa*, Berkeley, California University Press, 1992

Field, M., 'Mental Disorder in Rural Ghana', *The Journal of Mental Science*, 104, 1958, pp. 1043–51

Field, M.J., *Search for Security: An Ethno-Psychiatric Study of Rural Ghana*, Evanston, IL, Northwestern University Press, 1960

Fildes, Valerie, Lara Marks and Hilary Marland (eds.), *Women and Children First: International Maternal and Infant Welfare, 1870–1945*, London, Routledge, 1992

Foster, W.D., *The Church Missionary Society and Modern Medicine in Uganda the Life of Sir Albert Cook, K.C.M.G., 1870–1951*, Newhaven, Newhaven Press,1978

Foster, W.D., *The Early History of Scientific Medicine in Uganda*, Nairobi, East African Literature Bureau, 1970

Foster, W.D., 'Robert Moffat and the Beginnings of the Government Medical Service in Uganda', *Medical History*, 13, 1969, pp. 237–50

Foster, W.D., 'Doctor Albert Cook and the Early Days of the Church Missionary Society's Medical Mission to Uganda', *Medical History*, 12, 4, 1968, pp. 325–43

Geber, M., 'The Psycho-Motor Development of African Children in the First Year, and the Influence of Maternal Behavior', *Journal of Social Psychology*, 47, 1958, pp. 185–95

Geber, M. and R. Dean, 'Psychological Factors in the Etiology of Kwashiorkor', *Bulletin of the World Health Organization*, 12, 3, 1955, pp. 471–5

Gelfand, Michael, *A Service to the Sick: A History of the Health Services for Africans in Southern Rhodesia, 1890–1953*, Gweru, Mambo Press, 1976

Gelfand, Michael, *Tropical Victory: An Account of the Influence of Medicine on the History of Southern Rhodesia, 1900–1923*, Cape Town, Juta, 1953

Ghai, Dharam P. and Yash P. Ghai (eds.), *Portrait of a Minority: Asians in East Africa*, Nairobi and London, Oxford University Press, 1970

Gilbert, Erik, *Dhows and the Colonial Economy in Zanzibar: 1860–1970*, Oxford, James Currey, 2004

Gilks, John Langton, 'The Medical Department and the Health Organization of Kenya, 1909–1933', *The East African Medical Journal*, 9, 1932–3, pp. 340–54

Gish, Oscar, 'Color and Skill: British Immigration, 1955–68', *International Migration Review*, 3, 1968, pp. 19–37

Glassman, Jonathon, 'Slower than a Massacre: The Multiple Sources of Racial Thought in Colonial Africa', *American Historical Review*, 109, 2004, pp. 720–54

Glassman, Jonathon, 'Sorting out the Tribes: The Creation of Racial Identities in Colonial Zanzibar's Newspaper Wars', *Journal of African History*, 41, 2000, pp. 395–428

Good, Charles, *The Steamer Parish: The Rise and Fall of Missionary Medicine on an African Frontier*, London, University of Chicago Press, 2004

Gopal, M., D. Balasubramanian, P. Kanagarajah, A. Anirudhan and P. Murugan, 'Madras Medical College, 175 Years of Medical Heritage', *The National Medical Journal of India*, 23, 2, 2010, pp. 117–20

Gordon, H., 'The Mental Capacity of the African', *Journal of the Royal African Society*, 33, 1934, pp. 226–42

Grant, Kevin, Philippa Levine and Frank Trentmann (eds.), *Beyond Sovereignty, 1880–1950: Britain, Empire and Transnationalism*, London, Palgrave, 2007

Greenwood, Anna and Harshad Topiwala, *Indian Doctors in Kenya: The Forgotten Story, 1895–1940*, London, Palgrave Macmillan, 2015

Gregory, Robert G., *India and East Africa: A History of Race Relations within the British Empire, 1890–1939*, Oxford, Clarendon Press, 1971

Guha, Ranajit, 'The Small Voice of History', in Shahid Amin and Dipesh Chakrabarty (eds.), *Subaltern Studies: Writings on South Asian History and Society*, Vol. IX, Oxford, Oxford University Press, 1988, pp. 1–12

Hailey, A., *An African Survey. A Study of Problems arising in Africa, South of the Sahara*, 2nd edn, Oxford, Oxford University Press, 1957

Hammond, D. and A. Jablow, *The Africa that Never Was: Four Centuries of British Writing about Africa*, New York, Twayne, 1970

Hardiman, David, *Missionaries and their Medicine: A Christian Modernity for Tribal India*, Manchester, New York, Manchester University Press, 2008

Hardiman, David (ed.), *Healing Bodies, Saving Souls: Medical Missions in Asia and Africa*, Amsterdam and New York, Rodopi, 2006

Hardiman, David and Projit Mukharji (eds.), *Medical Marginality in South Asia: Situating Subaltern Therapeutics*, London, Routledge, 2012

Harris, T., *Donkey's Gratitude: Twenty-two Years in the Growth of a New African Nation – Tanzania*, Durham, Pentland Press, 1992

Harrison, Mark, *Public Health in British India: Anglo-Indian Preventative Medicine 1859–1914*, Cambridge, Cambridge University Press, 1994

Hartwig, Friedhelm, 'The Segmentation of the Indian Ocean Region. Arabs and the Implementation of Immigration Regulations in Zanzibar and British East Africa', in Jan-Georg Deutsch and Brigitte Reinwald (eds.), *Space on the Move. Transformations of the Indian Ocean Seascape in the Nineteenth and Twentieth Century*, Berlin, Klaus Schwarz Verlag, 2002, pp. 21–35

Hastings, A., *Christian Marriage in Africa, Being a Report Commissioned by the Archbishops of Cape Town, Central Africa, Kenya, Tanzania, and Uganda*, London, SPCK, 1973

Haynes, Douglas M., 'Framing Tropical Disease in London: Patrick Manson, *Filaria Perstans*, and the Uganda Sleeping Sickness Epidemic, 1891–1902', *Social History of Medicine*, 13, 3, 2000, pp. 467–93

Headrick, Daniel R., *The Tools of Empire: Technology and European Imperialism in the Nineteenth Century*, Oxford, Oxford University Press, 1981

Healy, David, *Let Them Eat Prozac: The Unhealthy Relationship between the Pharmaceutical Industry and Depression*, New York, New York University Press, 2004

Heaton, Matthew M., 'Stark Roving Mad: The Repatriation of Nigerian Mental Patients and the Global Construction of Mental Illness, 1906–1960', unpublished PhD thesis, University of Texas at Austin, 2008

Henin, R., *National Demographic Survey of Tanzania, 1973: Volume II, Data for Socioeconomic Groups*, Dar es Salaam, Tanzania Bureau of Statistics, 1973

Herbert, Eugenia W., 'Smallpox Inoculation in Africa', *Journal of African History*, 16, 4, 1975, pp. 539–59

Hodges, Sarah, *Contraception, Colonialism and Commerce: Birth Control in South India, 1920–1940*, Aldershot, Ashgate, 2008

Hokkanen, Markku, *Medicine and Scottish Missionaries in the Northern Malawi Region: Quests for Health in a Colonial Society*, Lewiston, The Edwin Mellen Press, 2007

Hollingsworth, Lawrence William, *The Asians of East Africa*, London, Macmillan and Co. Ltd., 1960

Hoppe, Kirk Arden, *Lords of the Fly: Sleeping Sickness Control in British East Africa, 1900–1960*, Westport, CT, Praeger, 2003

Hudson, Nicholas, 'From "Nation" to "Race": The Origin of Racial Classification in Eighteenth-Century Thought', *Eighteenth- Century Studies*, 29, 1996, pp. 247–64

Hunt, N., *A Colonial Lexicon of Birth Ritual, Medicalization and Mobility in the Congo*, Durham NC, Duke University Press, 1999

Huxley, E., *The Sorcerer's Apprentice*, London, Chatto and Windus, 1948

Iliffe, J., *East African Doctors*, Cambridge, Cambridge University Press, 1998

Jackson, Lynette, *Surfacing Up: Psychiatry and Social Order in Colonial Zimbabwe, 1908–1968*, Ithaca, NY, Cornell University Press, 2005

Janzen, John M., *The Quest for Therapy in Lower Zaire*, Berkeley, University of California Press, 1978

Jeffries, Charles, *Partners for Progress: The Men and Women of the Colonial Service*, London, George G. Harrap, 1949

Jeffries, Charles, *The Colonial Empire and its Civil Service*, Cambridge, Cambridge University Press, 1938

Jelliffe, D., 'Custom and Child Health I', *Tropical and Geographical Medicine*, 15, 1963, pp. 121–3

Jelliffe, D., 'Village Level Feeding of Young Children in Developing Tropical Regions, with Especial Reference to Buganda', *Journal of the American Medical Women's Association*, 17, 5 May 1962, pp. 409–18

Jelliffe, D. 'The Need for Health Education', Report of a Seminar on Health Education and the Mother and Child in East Africa', Makerere Medical School, Kampala, November 1961

Jelliffe, D., H. Welbourn and F. Bennett, 'Child Rearing and Personal Development in Africa', unpublished typescript in the possession of Hebe Welbourn, n.d. [c.1961]

Jennings, Michael, 'Common Counsel, Common Policy: Healthcare, Missions and the Rise of the "Voluntary Sector" in Colonial Tanzania', *Development and Change*, 44, 4, 2013, pp. 939–63

Jennings, Michael, '"Healing of Bodies, Salvation of Souls": Missionary Medicine in Colonial Tanganyika, 1870s-1939', *Journal of Religion in Africa* 38, 2008, pp. 27–56

Jennings, Michael, '"A Matter of Vital Importance": The Place of Medical Mission in Maternal and Child Healthcare in Tanganyika, 1919–39', in David Hardiman (ed.), *Healing Bodies, Saving Souls: Medical Missions in Asia and Africa*, Amsterdam and New York, Rodopi, 2006, pp. 227–50

Jennings, Michael, '"This Mysterious and Intangible Enemy": Health and Disease amongst the Early UMCA Missionaries, 1860–1918', *Social History of Medicine*, 15, 1, 2002, pp. 65–87

Joalahliae, Randolph M.K., *The Indian as an Enemy: An Analysis of the Indian Question in East Africa*, Bloomington, IN, Authorhouse, 2010

Johnson, Ryan, '*Mantsemei*, Interpreters and the Successful Eradication of Plague: The 1908 Plague Epidemic in Colonial Accra', in Ryan Johnson and Amna Khalid (eds.), *Public Health in the British Empire: Intermediaries, Subordinates, and the Practice of Public Health, 1850–1960*, New York, Routledge, 2012

Johnson, Ryan, 'Colonial Mission and Imperial Tropical Medicine: Livingstone College, London, 1893–1914', *Social History of Medicine*, 23, 3, 2010, pp. 49–66

Johnson, Ryan, '"An All-White Institution": Defending Private Practice and the Formation of the West African Medical Staff', *Medical History*, 54, 2010, pp. 237–54

Johnson, Ryan, 'The West African Medical Staff and the Administration of Imperial Tropical Medicine, 1902–14', *The Journal of Imperial and Commonwealth History*, 38, 3, 2010, pp. 419–39

Johnson, Ryan and Amna Khalid (eds.), *Public Health in the British Empire: Intermediaries, Subordinates, and the Practice of Public Health*, New York and London, Routledge, 2012

Johnston, H., *The Uganda Protectorate*, London, Hutchinson, 1902

Jones, Margaret, *Health Policy in Britain's Model Colony: Ceylon (1900–1948)*, New Delhi, Orient Longman, 2004

Kaggwa, A., *The Customs of the Baganda*, trans. E. Kalibala, ed. M. Edel, New York, Columbia University Press, 1934

Kalusa, Walima T., 'Language, Medical Auxiliaries, and the Re-interpretation of Missionary Medicine in Colonial Mwinilunga, Zambia, 1922–51', *Journal of Eastern African Studies*, 1, 1, 2007, pp. 57–78

Keller, Richard C., *Colonial Madness: Psychiatry in French North Africa*, Chicago, University of Chicago Press, 2007

Kennedy, Dane and Durba Ghosh (eds.), *Decentring Empire: Britain, India, and the Transcolonial World*, New Delhi, Longman Orient Press, 2006

Kidd, Cecil B., 'Psychiatric Morbidity among Students', *British Journal of Preventive and Social Medicine*, 19, 1965, p. 143–50

King, Michael and King, Elspeth, *The Story of Medicine and Disease in Malawi: The 150 Years Since Livingstone*, Blantyre, The Montfort Press, 1997

Kirk-Greene, Anthony, *Britain's Imperial Administrators, 1858–1966*, London, Macmillan, 2000

Kirk-Greene, Anthony, *On Crown Service: A History of HM Colonial and Overseas Civil Services, 1837–1997*, London, I.B. Tauris, 1999

Kirk-Greene, Anthony, *A Biographical Dictionary of the British Colonial Service, 1939–1966*, London, H. Zell, 1991

Kirk-Greene, Anthony, 'The Thin White Line: The Size of the British Colonial Service in Africa', *African Affairs*, 79, 1980, pp. 25–44

Koku, M. and M. Ngaiza, 'The Life History of a Housewife: Her Life, Work, Income and Property Ownership', in M. Ngaiza and B. Koda (eds.), *Unsung Heroines: Women's Life Histories from Tanzania*, Dar es Salaam, WRDP, 1991, pp. 85–108

Kollman, P., *The Victoria Nyanza: The Land, the Races and their Customs, with Specimens of Some of the Dialects*, London, Swan Sonnenschein, 1899

Kuhanen, Jan, *Poverty, Health and Reproduction in Early Colonial Uganda*, Joensuu, Finland, University of Joensuu Publications in the Humanities, 37, 2005

Kuper, A., *Anthropology and Anthropologists: The Modern British School*, London, Routledge & Kegan Paul, 1983

Kyle, Keith, 'Gandhi, Harry Thuku and Early Kenya Nationalism', *Transition*, 27, 1966, pp. 16–22

Laidlaw, Zoe, *Colonial Connections 1815–45; Patronage, the Information Revolution and Colonial Government*, Manchester, Manchester University Press, 2005

Lakoff, Andrew, *Pharmaceutical Reason: Knowledge and Value in Global Psychiatry*, Cambridge, Cambridge University Press, 2005

Langwick, Stacey, *Bodies, Politics and African Healing: The Matter of Maladies in Tanzania*, Bloomington, Indiana University Press, 2011

Larsson, B., *Conversion to Greater Freedom? Women, Church and Social Change in North-Western Tanzania under Colonial Rule*, Uppsala, University of Uppsala, 1991

Lasker, Judith N., 'The Role of Health Services in Colonial Rule: the Case of the Ivory Coast', *Culture, Medicine and Psychiatry*, 1, 1977, pp. 277–97

Laurie, W., 'A Pilot Scheme of Venereal Disease Control in East Africa', *British Journal of Venereal Diseases*, 34 1958, pp. 16–21

Laurie, W. and H. Trant, *East African Medical Survey, Monograph no. 2: A Health Survey in Bukoba District, Tanganyika*, Nairobi, EAHC, 1954

Lawrance, Benjamin, N., Emily Lynn Osborn and Richard L. Roberts (eds.), *Intermediaries, Interpreters, and Clerks: African Employees in the Making of Colonial Africa*, Madison, University of Wisconsin Press, 2006

Lejju, B., P. Robertshaw and D. Taylor, 'Africa's Earliest Bananas?', *Journal of Archaeological Science*, 33, 1 2006, pp. 102–13

Lester, Alan, 'Imperial Circuits and Networks: Geographies of the British Empire', *History Compass*, 4, 2006, pp. 124–41

Lester, Alan, *Imperial Networks: Creating Identities in Nineteenth-Century South Africa and Britain*, London, Routledge, 2001

Littlewood, Roland, and Maurice Lipsedge, *Aliens and Alienists: Ethnic Minorities and Psychiatry*, New York, Penguin, 1982

Livingston, Julie, *Debility and the Moral Imagination in Botswana*, Bloomington, Indiana University Press, 2005

Lloyd-Jones, W., *K.A.R.: Being an Unofficial Account of the Origin and Activities of the King's African Rifles*, London, Arrowsmith, 1926

Lloyd-Jones, W., *Havash Frontier Adventures in Kenya*, London, Arrowsmith, 1925

Lonsdale, J., 'Mau Maus of the Mind: Making Mau Mau and Remaking Kenya', *Journal of African History*, 31, 3, 1990, pp. 393–421

Lugard, F., *The Dual Mandate in British Tropical Africa*, Edinburgh, Blackwood, 1922

Lwanda, John, 'Politics, Culture and Medicine in Malawi: Historical Continuities and Ruptures with Special Reference to HIV/AIDS', unpublished PhD thesis, University of Edinburgh, 2002

Lyons, Maryinez, *The Colonial Disease: A Social History of Sleeping Sickness in Northern Zaire 1900–1940*, Cambridge, Cambridge University Press, 2002 [first published, 1992]

Lyons, Maryinez, 'The Power to Heal: African Medical Auxiliaries in Colonial Belgian Congo and Uganda', in Dagmar Engels and Shula Marks (eds.), *Contesting Colonial Hegemony: State and Society in Africa and India*, London, British Academic Press, 1994, 202–23.

McCracken, John, *Politics and Christianity in Malawi: The Impact of the Livingstonia Mission in the Northern Province*, Blantyre, CLAIM, 2000

McCracken, John, 'Experts and Expertise in Colonial Malawi', *African Affairs*, 81, 1982, pp. 101–16

McCulloch, J., *Colonial Psychiatry and 'The African Mind'*, Cambridge, Cambridge University Press, 1995

McGregor, J. and T. Ranger, 'Displacement and Disease: Epidemics and Ideas about Malaria in Matabeleland, Zimbabwe, 1945–1996', *Past and Present*, 167, 2000, pp. 203–38

McKelvey Jr, J.J., *Man Against Tsetse: Struggle for Africa*, London, Cornell University Press, 1973

Macleod, Roy and Milton Lewis (eds.), *Disease Medicine and Empire*, London, Routledge, 1988

McMaster, D., 'Change of Regional Balance in the Bukoba district of Tanganyika', *Tanganyika Notes and Records*, 56 1961, pp. 79–92

Madeira, Ana, 'Portuguese, French and British Discourses on Colonial Education: Church–State Relations, School Expansion and Missionary Competition in Africa, 1890–1930', *Paedagogica Historica* 41, 1/2, 2005, pp. 31–60

Mahone, Sloan and Megan Vaughan (eds.), *Psychiatry and Empire*, New York, Palgrave Macmillan, 2007

Mair, L., *An African People in the Twentieth Century*, London, Routledge, 1934

Manchuelle, Francois, *Willing Migrants: Soninke Labor Diasporas, 1848–1960*, Athens, Ohio University Press, 1997

Mangan, James Anthony, *'Benefits Bestowed'? Education and British Imperialism*, Manchester University Press, 1988

Mangat, J.S., *A History of the Asians in East Africa, c.1886–1945*, Oxford, Oxford University Press, 1969

Martin, C.J., 'A Demographic Study of an Immigrant Community: The Indian Population of British East Africa', *Population Studies*, 6.3, 1953, pp. 233–47

Maxon, R.M., *Struggle for Kenya: The Loss and Reassertion of Imperial Initiative, 1912–1923*, London, Fairleigh Dickinson University Press, 1993

McCracken, John, *A History of Malawi*, Woodbridge, James Currey, 2012

Metcalf, T.M., *Imperial Connections: India in the Indian Ocean Arena, 1860–1920*, Berkeley and London, University of California Press, 2007

Midgley, James and David Piachaud (eds.), *Colonialism and Welfare: Social Policy and the British Imperial Legacy*, London, Edward Elgar Publishing, 2012

Milne, Arthur Dawson, 'The Rise of the Colonial Medical Service', *Kenya and East African Medical Journal*, 5, 1928–9, pp. 50–8

Milne, G., 'Bukoba: High and Low Fertility on a Laterised soil', *The East African Agricultural Journal*, 4, 1938, pp. 1–21

Morgan, Philip D. and Sean Hawkins (eds.), *Black Experience and the Empire*, Oxford, Oxford University Press, 2004

Mtawali, C., 'A Health Campaign in Tanganyika Territory', *Community Development Bulletin*, 2, 1951, pp. 54–6

Mungeam, G.H., *Kenya: Select Historical Documents 1884–1923*, Nairobi, East African Publishing House, 1979

Muraleedharan, V.R., 'Professionalising Medical Practice in Colonial South India', *Economic and Political Weekly*, 27, 4, 1992, pp. PE27–30

Nair, T.D., 'A Tana River Yaws Campaign', *Kenya and East Africa Medical Journal*, 1927, pp. 201–7

Neill, Deborah J., *Networks in Tropical Medicine: Internationalism, Colonialism, and the Rise of a Medical Specialty, 1890–1930*, Stanford, Stanford University Press, 2012

Nichols, S., *Red Strangers: The White Tribes of Kenya*, London, Timewell Press, 2005

Oliver, Ronald, *The Missionary Factor in East Africa*, London, Longmans, 1952

Olukoju, Ayodeji, 'Imperial Business Umpire: The Colonial Office, United Africa Company, Elder Dempster, and "The Great Shipping War" of 1929–1930', in Toyin Falola and Emily Brownell (eds.), *Africa, Empire and Globalization: Essays in Honor of A.G. Hopkins*, Durham, NC, Carolina Academic Press, 2011, pp. 167–89

Olukoju, Ayodeji, '"Helping Our Own Shipping": Official Passages to Nigeria, 1914–45', *Journal of Transport History*, 20, 1999, pp. 30–45

Olukoju, Ayodeji, 'Elder Dempster and the Shipping Trade of Nigeria during the First World War', *Journal of African History*, 33, 1992, pp. 255–71

Owens, Geoffrey Ross, 'Exploring the Articulation of Governmentality and Sovereignty: The Chwaka Road and the Bombardment of Zanzibar', *Journal of Colonialism and Colonial History*, 8, 2007, pp. 1–55

Oza, Uchhrangrai Keshavrai, *The Rift in the Empire's Lute: Being a History of the Indian Struggle in Kenya from 1900 to 1930*, Nairobi, Advocate of India Press, 1930

Packard, Randall, *White Plague, Black Labor: Tuberculosis and the Political Economy of Health and Disease in South Africa*, Berkeley, University of California Press, 1989

Paice, Edward, *Lost Lion of Empire: The Life of 'Cape to Cairo' Grogan*, London, Harper Collins, 2001

Parkinson, Cosmo, *The Colonial Office from Within, 1909–1945*, London, Faber and Faber Ltd., 1947

Parle, Julie, 'The Fools on the Hill: The Natal Government Asylum and the Institutionalisation of Insanity in Colonial Natal', *Journal of Natal and Zulu History*, 19, 2001, pp. 1–40

Pashid, Abdur, *History of the King Edward Medical College Lahore, 1860–1960*, Lahore, King Edward Medical College, 1960

Pati, Biswamoy and Mark Harrison (eds.), *The Social History of Health and Medicine in Colonial India*, London and New York, Routledge, 2009

Patton, Adell, *Physicians, Colonial Racism and Diaspora in West Africa*, Gainesville, University of Florida Press, 1996

Pearson, M.N., *Port Cities and Intruders: The Swahili Coast, India and Portugal in the Early Modern Era*, Baltimore, Johns Hopkins University Press, 1998

Porter, Andrew, '"Cultural imperialism" and Protestant Missionary Enterprise, 1780–1914', *Journal of Imperial and Commonwealth History*, 25, 3, 1997, pp. 367–91

Potter, Simon J., 'Webs, Networks and Systems: Globalization and the Mass

Media in the Nineteenth- and Twentieth-Century British Empire', *Journal of British Studies*, 46, 2007, pp. 621–46

Prince, Raymond, 'The "Brain Fag" Syndrome in Nigerian Students', *Journal of Mental Science*, 106, 1960, pp. 559–70

Pringle, Yolana, 'Investigating "Mass Hysteria" in Early Postcolonial Uganda: Benjamin H. Kagwa, East African Psychiatry, and the Gisu', *Journal of the History of Medicine and Allied Sciences*, 70, 1, 2015, pp. 105–36

Prior, C., *Exporting Empire: Africa, Colonial Officials and the Construction of the British Imperial State, c.1900–39*, Manchester, Manchester University Press, 2013

Rafferty, Anne-Marie, 'The Rise and Demise of the Colonial Nursing Service: British Nurses in the Colonies, 1896–1966', *Nursing History Review*, 15, 2007, pp. 147–54

Ramanna, Mridula, *Western Medicine and Public Health in Colonial Bombay, 1845–1895*, Delhi, Orient Longman, 2002

Ramanna, Mridula, 'Indian Doctors, Western Medicine and Social Change, 1845–1885', in Mariam Dossal and Ruby Maloni (eds.), *State Intervention and Popular Response: Western India in the Nineteenth Century*, Mumbai, Popular Prakashan, 1999, pp. 40–62

Ranger, T., 'Godly Medicine: The Ambiguities of Medical Mission in Southeastern Tanzania, 1900–1945', in S. Feierman and John M Janzen (eds.), *The Social Basis of Health and Healing in Africa*, Berkeley, Los Angeles and Oxford, University of California Press, 1992, pp. 256–82

Rehse, H., *Kiziba: Land und Leute*, Stuttgart, Strecker und Schröder, 1910

Reining, P., 'The Haya: The Agrarian System of a Sedentary People', unpublished PhD dissertation, University of Chicago, 1967

Reining, P. and A. Richards, 'Report on Fertility Surveys in Buganda and Buhaya, 1952', in F. Lorimer et al. (eds.), *Culture and Human Fertility*, Paris, UNESCO, 1954, pp. 351–404

Rennick, Agnes, 'Church and Medicine: The Role of Medical Missionaries in Malawi 1875–1914', unpublished PhD thesis, University of Stirling, 2003

Richards, A., *The Changing Structure of a Ganda Village: Kisozi, 1892–1952*, Nairobi, EAPH, 1966

Richards, A., 'Traditional Values and Current Political Behavior', in L. Fallers, (ed.) *All The King's Men: Leadership and Status in Buganda on the Eve of Independence*, London, Oxford University Press, 1964, pp. 294–335

Richards, A., *Land, Labour, and Diet in Northern Rhodesia: An Economic Study of the Bemba Tribe*, Oxford, Oxford University Press, 1939

Roscoe, J., *The Baganda: An Account of Their Native Customs and Beliefs*, London, Macmillan, 1911

Ross, Andrew C., *Blantyre Mission and the Making of Modern Malawi*, Blantyre, CLAIM, 1996

Ross, W.G., *Kenya from Within: A Short Political History*, London, George Allen, 1927

Sadowsky, Jonathan, *Imperial Bedlam: Institutions of Madness in Colonial Southwest Nigeria*, Berkeley, University of California Press, 1999

Salvadori, Cynthia, *We Came in Dhows*, Nairobi, Paperchase Kenya Ltd, 1996

Schoenbrun, D., 'Cattle Herds and Banana Gardens: The Historical Geography of the Western Great Lakes Region, ca AD 800–1500', *The African Archaeological Review*, 11, 1993, pp. 39–72

Schram, Ralph, *A History of the Nigerian Health Services*, Ibadan, Ibadan University Press, 1971

Sen, S.N., *Scientific and Technical Education in India 1781–1900*, New Delhi, Indian National Science Academy, 1991

Shannon, M., 'Rebuilding the Social Life of the Kikuyu', *African Affairs*, 56, 1957, pp. 272–84

Shelley, H. and W. Watson, 'An Investigation Concerning Mental Disorder in Nyasaland', *Jounral of Mental Science*, 82, 1936, pp. 701–30

Shepperson, George and Thomas Price Thomas, *Independent African*, Edinburgh, Edinburgh University Press, 1958

Sheriff, Abdul, 'The Spatial Dichotomy of Swahili Towns: The Case of Zanzibar in the Nineteenth Century', *Azania*, 67, 2002, pp. 63–81

Sheriff, Abdul, *Slaves, Spices and Ivory in Zanzibar: Integration of an East African Commercial Empire into the World Economy, 1770–1873*, London, James Currey, 1987

Sherwood, Marika, 'African Seamen, Elder Dempster and the Government, 1940–42', *Immigrants and Minorities*, 13, 1994, pp. 30–45

Sherwood, Marika, 'Elder Dempster and West Africa 1891–c.1940: The Genesis of Underdevelopment', *International Journal of African Historical Studies*, 30, 1993, pp. 253–76

Shumaker, L., *Africanizing Anthropology: Fieldwork, Networks, and the Making of Cultural Knowledge in Central Africa*, Durham NC, Duke University Press, 2001

Smith, Edwin W., *The Christian Mission in Africa: A Study Based on the Proceedings of the International Conference at Le Zoute, Belgium, September 14th to 21st, 1926*, London, International Missionary Council, 1926

Smith, John (ed.), *Administering Empire: The British Colonial Service in Retrospect*, University of London Press, 1999

Sorenson, M., *Land Reform in the Kikuyu Country*, Nairobi, Oxford University Press, 1967

Sorrenson, M.P.K., *Origin of European Settlement in Kenya*, London, Oxford University Press, 1968

Southall, A. and P. Gutkind, *Townsmen in the Making: Kampala and Its Suburbs*, Kampala, EAISR, 1957

Squires, H.C., *The Sudan Medical Service: An Experiment in Social Medicine*, London, William Heinemann, 1958

Stanley, Brian, *The Bible and the Flag: Protestant Missions and British Imperialism in the Nineteenth and Twentieth Centuries*, Leicester, Apollos, 1990

Still, R.J., 'Mental Health in Overseas Students', *Proceedings of the British Student Health Association*, 1961, pp. 59–61

Summers, C., 'Radical Rudeness: Ugandan Social Critiques in the 1940s', *Journal of Social History*, 39, 3, 2006, pp. 741–70

Summers, Carol, 'Intimate Colonialism: The Imperial Production of Reproduction in Uganda, 1907–1925', *Signs*, 16, 4, 1991, pp. 787–807

Tappan, J., '"A Healthy Child Comes from a Healthy Mother": Mwanamugimu and Nutritional Science in Uganda, 1935–1973', unpublished PhD dissertation, Columbia University, 2010

Tilley, H., *Africa as a Living Laboratory: Empire, Development, and the Problem of Scientific Knowledge, 1870–1950*, Chicago, University of Chicago Press, 2011

Titmuss, R.M., *The Health Services of Tanganyika: A Report to the Government*, London, Pitman Medical Publishing Co., 1964

Tooth, Geoffrey, *Studies in Mental Illness in the Gold Coast*, London, His Majesty's Stationery Office, 1950

Trowell, H.C., 'The Medical Pioneers and Explorers of East Africa', *East African Medical Journal*, 34, 8, 1957, pp. 417–30

Trowell, H. et al., *Kwashiorkor*, 2nd edn, London, 1982

Tuck, Michael William, 'Syphilis, Sexuality, and Social Control: A History of Venereal Disease in Colonial Uganda', unpublished PhD thesis, Northwestern University, 1997

Turshen, B., 'The Impact of Colonialism on Health and Health Services in Tanzania', *International Journal of Health Services* 7, 1977, pp. 7–35

van Tol, Deanne, 'Mothers, Babies, and the Colonial State: The Introduction of Maternal and Infant Welfare Services in Nigeria, 1925–1945', *Spontaneous Generations*, 1, 2007, pp. 110–31

Vaughan, Megan, *Curing Their Ills: Colonial Power and African Illness*, Cambridge, Polity Press, 1991

Vaughan, Megan, 'Idioms of Madness: Zomba Lunatic Asylum, Nyasaland, in the Colonial Period', *Journal of Southern African Studies*, 9, 1983, pp. 218–38

Vongsathorn, Kathleen, '"First and Foremost the Evangelist"? Mission and Government Priorities for the Treatment of Leprosy in Uganda, 1927–48', *Journal of Eastern African Studies*, 6, 3, 2012, pp. 544–60

Watts, M., *Silent Violence: Food, Famine and Peasantry in Northern Nigeria*, Berkeley, University of California Press, 1983

Welbourn, H., 'Weaning among the Baganda', *Journal of Tropical Pediatrics*, 9, 1 1963, pp. 14–24

Welbourn, H., 'Backgrounds and Follow-up of Children with Kwashiorkor', *Journal of Tropical Paediatrics*, 5, 4, 1959, pp. 84–95

Welbourn, H., 'The Danger Period during Weaning. A Study of Baganda Children Who Were Attending Child Welfare Clinics near Kampala, Uganda', unpublished MD dissertation, University of Birmingham, 1952

Williams, Audrey W., 'The History of Mulago Hospital and the Makerere College Medical School', *East African Medical Journal*, 29, 1952, pp. 253–63

Williams, C., 'Kwashiorkor: A Nutritional Disease of Children Associated with a Maize Diet', *Lancet*, 16 November 1935, pp. 1151–2

[191]

Worboys, Michael, 'The Colonial World as Mission and Mandate: Leprosy and Empire, 1900–1940', *Osiris*, 15, 2000, pp. 207–18

Worboys, M., 'The Discovery of Colonial Malnutrition Between the Wars', in D. Arnold (ed.), *Imperial Medicine and Indigenous Societies*, Manchester, Manchester University Press, 1988, pp. 208–25

Wylie, Diana, 'Confrontation over Kenya: The Colonial Office and Its Critics, 1918–1940', *Journal of African History*, 18.3, 1977, pp. 427–47

Youé, Christopher P., 'The Threat of Settler Rebellion and the Imperial Predicament: The Denial of Indian Rights in Kenya, 1923', *Canadian Journal of History*, 12, 1978, pp. 347–60

Young, W., 'Extra-urethritic Cases in an African Venereal Diseases Hospital', *The British Journal of Venereal Diseases*, 20 1944, pp. 151–4

Younghusband, Ethel, *Glimpses of East Africa and Zanzibar*, London, John Long, 1910

Zeller, Diane L., 'The Establishment of Western Medicine in Buganda', unpublished PhD thesis, Columbia University, 1971

INDEX

Africa Inland Mission 158, 160, 163
African dressers 66, 78–9
    see also dressers
African Medical Assistants 20, 29, 45
Ainsworth, John 67, 143
Ainsworth, Mary 142–3
anthropologists 13, 33, 110, 112, 127,
        132, 137, 141–2, 144
    see also anthropologists;
        ethnographers; ethnography
anthropology 132
    see also anthropologists;
        ethnographers; ethnography
Arabs 3, 12, 66, 85–9, 92, 94–100
Assistant Surgeon 12, 64, 68–71, 78

Belfield, Henry 73, 75
Belgian Congo 46–7, 157
Bennett, Frank 143
Beveridge, William 130
bilharzia 52
Blantyre
    mission 40–1, 43–5, 47, 54, 57
    town 39, 41–3, 45, 48, 53, 55, 57–8
Bond, Ashton 24–7
Bowlby, John 141
Bowring, Charles 73
Bowring Report (1922) 65, 73–5, 77,
        79
    see also Economic and Finance
        Committee Report (1922)
British Central Africa Protectorate
        40–1
    see also Malawi; Nyasaland
British Medical Association (BMA)
        8, 23, 77
Bruce, David 47
Buganda 13, 28–9, 126, 137–9, 142–6
    see also Ganda
Buhaya 13, 126–37, 144–6
    see also Haya

Calcutta Medical College 68
Carothers, J.C. 111
cataract 58
Central Midwives Board 52
cerebro-spinal meningitis 25
Chamberlain, Joseph 4–5
Cheonga, Thomas 53
child health 93, 97, 140, 143, 146,
        158, 166
Chilembwe Rising 44, 55
Chisholm, James 46–7, 50
Christian Council of Tanganyika
        160–1, 163
Church Missionary Society (CMS)
        11, 19–32, 158, 160–2
Church of Scotland 40–1, 56
Clearkin, Peter 71
Colonial Office 4–5, 7–8, 12–13,
        15, 43, 56–7, 76, 93, 107, 112,
        114–17, 119–21, 127
Conference of Missionary Societies
        in Great Britain 56
constructive imperialism 4
Cook, Albert Ruskin 20–3, 29–31, 34
Cook, Ernest, 24, 27, 29–30
Cook, Jack 22–3, 31
Cory, Hans 132–3, 135–7
Cross, David Kerr 43
Culwick, Arthur 132–3, 135–7
Culwick, Geraldine 132–3, 135–7

Davies, J.N.P. 139
de Boer, Henry 55–7, 59
deculturation 111
Delamere, Hugh Cholmondeley 73
detribalisation 132
Devonshire White Paper (1923) 65,
        75, 79
dispensaries 9, 22, 26, 28, 43–4, 53,
        129, 136, 158–9, 162, 164–5
    see also dispensary